Order this book online at www.trafford.com
or email orders@trafford.com

Most Trafford titles are also available at major online book retailers.

Printed in the United States of America.

ISBN: 978-1-4907-4357-8 (sc)
ISBN: 978-1-4907-4359-2 (hc)
ISBN: 978-1-4907-4358-5 (e)

Library of Congress Control Number: 2014914120

*Trafford rev. 08/20/2014*

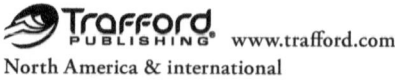 www.trafford.com

North America & international
toll-free: 1 888 232 4444 (USA & Canada)
fax: 812 355 4082

# MEDITATION:
## Deep Peace

Dennis Hill

# Table of Contents

# Preface

We will see the phrase *Deep Peace* throughout this volume; let us understand what this means in the context of the concepts presented. Deep Peace refers to the steady mental and emotional balance that is woven into every moment, in every circumstance, for all our life. Typically we cycle through a roller coaster of ups and downs, continuously reacting and recovering. This is only the mind caught up in its likes and dislikes, or worse. Just behind the mind, in the stillness of the watcher, is that serenity we seek. Only we don't know how to get free of this reactive inner voice.

Through meditation we begin to get glimpses of the stillness. With practice, the stillness enters us, and we begin to enjoy the spontaneous inner sense of serenity. Over time the stillness becomes the foundation of our perception and we look out on the world from our peaceful presence. Once we know this as our Self we can be free of the anxiety, doubt, disappointment, and fear, just being the watcher. This is Deep Peace.

It might come as a surprise that consciousness, the Self, is the watcher of the mind. In this we can become the impartial witness of mental dramas, creating separation between the watcher and the chaos of ego. Fortunately, the mind begins to like the stillness, and the suffering evaporates due to lack of interest. In this we become truly happy and content.

This volume will cover the cause of our suffering, lessons from the masters, and illumination of the final state of peace and bliss.

~Dennis Hill

# Introduction

Why do we do what we do? Isn't everything we do, ultimately, to bring us happiness? Think about it. All our planning, all our actions, all our manipulations, all our accumulations, are so that we can just be happy. When we get what we want, really, how long does it last? Is there a way that we can be happy all the time? The drive to fulfill our desires, in practice, does not bring us lasting happiness; so, what can we do?

*Satchidananda* is a Sanskrit term that describes the state of enduring happiness, and refers to the conscious substratum of existence. Let's break this down: *sat* is existence, or being; *chit* is consciousness, or sentiency; *ananda* is bliss, or enduring happiness. The traditional path to *satchidananda* that is taught in yoga philosophy (Advaita Vedanta) is simply the practice of meditation. In this practice we distill the inner caprice of thought down to simple stillness. As we get longer stretches of this stillness we become acquainted with the fullness of our essential being. In this fullness arises spontaneous joy, contentment and wisdom. This is the happiness that is always there in every moment. This book is a journal of clues along the way in the pursuit of enduring inner happiness, independent of outer circumstances—pleasurable or painful.

Bliss, according to Webster's Collegiate Dictionary, means "complete happiness." It derives from a German word that translates to "blithe:" a cheerful indifference. Why would one choose a path of complete happiness? Think about it! All our desires for things, people, wealth, influence, even the simple things in life, are ultimately to give us pleasure and make us happy. But bliss, as it turns out, is the very nature of our being. There is nothing we can possess, control, or accumulate that will bring us more happiness than just being immersed in transcendent self-awareness. Only we don't know this at the beginning. First, we must get all this stuff that should make us happy; then, we observe that everything changes over time, and the stuff we wanted causes us suffering in the end. What to do?

Most likely, we will just crave other stuff to see if that works out any better. Or, we could embark upon the adventurous search for what might bring happiness directly, without going through other stuff that brings us only to disappointment. As we go through life there are clues strewn along the path that point the way; it is up to us to seize upon these precious little pointers and see where they take us. We have to be very patient, yet persistent. If we do, there are glimpses of spontaneous joy that have actually been there all along. The path is just purifying the mind, so it no longer projects the veil of ignorance that hides the precious inner jewel of complete happiness.

There is one practice that is most essential in revealing the bliss of the Self—and that is meditation. This is the fundamental practice of mystics in all cultures that shows us the happiness that lies just behind the mind and shines its joyous radiance when the mind is at peace. If we can just spend some time every day in this sublime equanimity, we will get everything.

When I was eleven years old, my younger brother said to me, *I am going to have to be rich. I can't live any other way.* I thought this was remarkable, and promptly queried myself about what I wanted in my life to bring me happiness. It seemed the most likely candidate was to find the truth of everything. Now, a number of years down the road, my brother truly enjoys his personal wealth; and this is good. Likewise, my journey on the search for truth has been the most gratifying endeavor I can possibly imagine. There is a never-ending supply of mystery to apply this quizzical nature to, and the most arcane mystery holds the greatest thrill of the quest. It is just so gratifying that there is nothing that we have to take on faith; we can verify everything we are taught, in our own experience.

What is your interest in liberation, or even meditation for that matter? What does liberation even mean? It seems that people everywhere want liberation from something or other. There is political repression, family restriction, personal fear; so many thing that we want escape from. But how does meditation figure in with this concept of liberation? The inner stillness attained through this practice is liberation from the tyranny of the mind. The mind is a wonderful servant but an unforgiving tyrant. How do we break free from this lifetime of destructive and disturbing dramatics?

Only the mind suffers; so when the mind is quiet, the disturbance is forgotten. Suddenly we have peacefulness, contentment, and the pure joy of just being. This is the fullness of the emptiness. The more time we spend with this practice, the more we become immersed in the peaceful presence. Change comes gradually, but in the end we are free from suffering. Better than that, we live in the constant state of the silent witness, enjoying all that appears on the screen of life.

It is not necessary to withdraw from the world to follow this path less traveled by. Certainly we naturally turn inward as we go along, but we also follow *dharma* (doing the right thing), to live responsibly. Attaining liberation requires no effort because we are already enlightened—in the stillness just behind the mind. The effort is required in the restraint of the ego that will ultimately surrender to its true Self.

The topics presented here are entertainments for your mind with the hope that the substance that cannot be spoken will find its way to the light.

This work is organized in chronological order and is a simple compilation of notes to myself as I make my way through the years and through the fog of ignorance. It is a steady thread of inquiry over a number of years that has brought an enduring presence of peacefulness and a fullness of simple happiness.

~Dennis Hill

# *Dedication*

I dedicate this work to THIS;
beyond which there isn't, without which we aren't,
and within which the self-luminous Absolute
appears as the diversity.
This work is dedicated to the Guru,
who teaches us
through silence, service, grace and reverence
that our very being is the supracausal divine presence.
This work is dedicated to true love, serenity and delight,
that spontaneously emerges
when one is steady in the inner contentment.

# There Are So Many Questions!

*What Can I Do?*

If you are looking to calm the mind; the peaceful practice of meditation will allow you to be the observer of the mind's activities, thus becoming less involved in the urgency of emotional and mental drama. This practiced detachment is the first step toward the inner quiet where the mind becomes transparent to the inner equipoise that always lies just behind the mind. When the mind can be still, you will experience the pure happiness that is your true nature. As the practice of meditation matures, this inner serenity and balance will make its way into all corners of your life and you will be the happy and steady person on the outside that you truly are on the inside.

Meditation is an ancient tradition in all the world's cultures that has been practiced and taught for thousands of years by a few. If you are one of the few who would like to discover your inner Self and enjoy the happiness of your true nature, consider learning about the practice of meditation. If you can give yourself 15 minutes every day to sit quietly, it is certain that you will awaken the steady and cheerful person within.

*Levels of Meditation*

• **Learning About Meditation**

The student can learn, from a book or teacher, about the practice, purpose, and state of meditation without actually doing the practice.

• **Learning Meditation**

A book or teacher cannot teach the student meditation. Only meditation can teach meditation. It is in the actual practice that meditation is revealed.

- **Transcendence of the Mind**

Through the discipline of daily practice, one can glimpse the inner stillness that reveals the true Self of the meditator—consciousness itself, the impartial witness of the mind. In this stillness is the sweetness and serenity that exists continuously just behind the mind.

- **Attainment of the Steady State**

Over time, the meditator becomes established in the peaceful presence of the meditative state. The tyranny of the mind is overcome and one becomes free from a lifetime of mental conditioning. The meditator lives continuously in the happiness of the peaceful presence.

## Which Is Real; Waking or Dreaming?

I remember one morning in my seventh summer awakening after a particularly vivid dream. It seemed so real it caused me to wonder, Which is real, waking or dreaming? In my perplexity I went to my father (Dad has all the answers, right?) and asked him which is real. He said, "Waking is real; a dream can't be real because it's only a dream." From that, I knew that he didn't know the truth of the matter.

A story has been handed down about the great King Janaka of India. After a sumptuous meal in the courtyard of his palace, he lay down upon his canopied pallet to rest as his attendants fanned him, and his guards stood at the gate. Lying there, he fell into a dream that he was a thief and had been caught in the act of thievery and was being thrashed unmercifully. He awoke with a start and saw he was still the king and was being fanned by his servants and the guards were standing by the gate. With this comforting knowledge, he again dozed off and again found himself thrashed within an inch of his life. Again, he awoke to find himself a king being fanned by servants and guards standing by the gate. Determined to resolve the truth of the matter, he arose and called his court advisers and asked them, *which is real: waking or dreaming*.? None could give him a satisfactory answer, so he threw the lot of them in the dungeon.

It so happened that one of the advisers had a crippled son named Yajnavalkya who was an enlightened being; so, when his father did not come home that night, he inquired of his whereabouts and learned the story of the king's question. Thereupon, he presented himself to King Janaka who posed to the crippled boy his quandary. The boy told the king that neither waking nor dreaming was real. He said the only reality is a third state of consciousness which could only be attained through meditation, and to know the truth of all things that the king must become established in that state.

Voltaire has written, "When we dream we are dreaming, then we are very nearly awake." He too knew that in this waking dream we can awaken to consciousness beyond the mind, transcend the drama of the objective world and fantasy of the dream state, and live in the peace and joy of the one reality: the inner Self. This inner Self is witness to all other states and phenomena; this is the realm of inner peace and happiness.

## Just the Basics

One of the characteristics of life is consciousness. All life is conscious at some level of awareness according to its sophistication of sensory acuity. There is only one consciousness and each entity of life lives in this universal consciousness as well as in its local consciousness.

Human-kind has the highest potential for opening the field of universal consciousness fully into local consciousness. There are, however, many barriers to be overcome in the process and only few make any progress at all.

The first barrier is encountered soon after birth. That is, the local environment is so stimulating that the universal consciousness, being extremely subtle, is lost in the competition. Later, as language is learned, we fall under the spell of enchantment. We enter into the thralldom of the mind. The mind puts us to sleep.

It is only through stillness of mind that we begin to wake up again. In this stillness, the ecstasy of our true being flows into our lives. As one becomes established in stillness of mind, or witness consciousness, a re-centering takes place. We leave the anxieties of the made up drama and enter the unity of universal consciousness. Life in the world becomes a very high experience.

Amazing as it may seem, I have run across ancient literature that speak the truth of reality just as it is. As a sampling from the <u>Shiva Sutras</u> of Kashmir Shaivism, the first five sutras say it quite clearly:

1. The Self is consciousness.
2. Knowledge is bondage.
3. The sense of individuality of the empirical self is illusory. The sense of being the doer is illusory.
4. The words that arise in the mind are the basis of limited knowledge.
5. Right effort is staying in the awareness of universal consciousness.

Reading about it is one thing; mastery in stilling the mind is quite another. It appears that the mind is the disease of the Self. Enlightenment is to know the knower, hear the hearer, observe the observer.

Language is the fundamental neurosis of this species. The preoccupation with symbol-making arose as an adaptation to cope with sensory overload that came with crowding in early civilization 10,000 years ago. Our awareness has become dominated by symbolic laundering of sensory input and fantasy of past and future. This fabrication is the veil that corrupts the present reality and conceals the joyous tranquility of pristine consciousness.

To regain our full humanness, we must seek out the ecstasy of our being by stilling the ceaseless agitation of the mind. The suffering in our lives comes from believing that the made-up drama of words and pictures appearing in the mind is the reality. True happiness is found in becoming established in the state of consciousness unconditioned by the mind. This state is deep peace, divine bliss, Shiva, the peace that passeth understanding, Buddha nature, eternal life, Yoga, the absolute, and many other names for our original nature.

Once right understanding is attained, then suffering becomes optional, that is, a matter of choice. When one chooses pain over joy, it becomes almost comical that one would make such a choice, and the tragedy of it all begins to get diluted. Ultimately, we will cease allowing anything but the ecstasy of universal consciousness into our life. Really, happiness is what this life is all about. Finding the key to happiness is absolutely the greatest attainment of a lifetime.

There is not much else to say about it except that meditation is the path to enduring happiness.

## How Can We Awaken?

[Excerpt from a letter to Christine]

The great Sufi master Hazrat Inayat Khan has said: "The message is a call to those whose hour has come to awake, and it is a lullaby to those who are still meant to sleep."

If we are asleep, who or what is it that is supposed to awaken? Furthermore, what means are to be used to cause this awakening? From time to time, we all have inexplicable episodes of well-being, joy, even rapture. If we recognize this experience as an upwelling of our eternal nature and seek identity with this inner state, then we have set foot upon the path. Even if we have a great longing for we don't know what, it is this longing that is the driving force to reunite us with our lost Self, to re-member. The "I" who sleeps is the ego-self identified with the body and the play of incessant word pictures spun out by the mind. The

"I" who is fully awake is the eternal, unchanging, uncreated and undying, all knowing, all powerful and ever-present, the absolute, unconditioned consciousness. I, the eternal witness, observe myself patiently, dreaming the play.

The means: meditation. The Self sees through our eyes between the words. Awakening is remembering that I am the divine presence and I simply watch the play while being absorbed in the joyous tranquility of my true nature. In the beginning, of course, we are easily enthralled by the drama. But, gradually, the sweetness of our truest Self emerges and we drift free from the bondage of our limited self.

~

Meditation is a turning within, the opening of the inner eye, observing the observer. So, what do we see when we look in at what looks out, when we perceive that which perceives? We sense a live field of being, tangible to experience. It is formless, unbounded, not related to time and space, conscious, and intelligent. This is the silent witness of all manifestation. But, it is not as if the manifest is separate from the unmanifest. There is a force or driving power which streams through this conscious ground-state and creates light, thought, will, activity, knowledge, and feeling. This life stream is even audible as the inner sound. Out of the unmanifest is created the manifest aspects of the same unity. Throughout the ages, all who have sought the source find the same inner experience. We can only conclude that this sublime being of consciousness is the Self of all. So very gradual is the process of unfoldment. Much is required to overcome the conditioning of a lifetime. The teachings of the great beings bring the truth to the mind. The practice of meditation brings the truth of experience that the universe is consciousness and bliss. The subtle power of the true guru brings awakening and freedom: awakening to the true nature of our being, and freedom from the suffering caused by the tyranny of the mind. It is the teaching of Bhagwan Nityananda that:

*A person remains ordinary as long as he is led by the mind;*
*But, freed from the mind he becomes a great saint.*
*What is the use of many words?*
*Meditate.*
*You will get everything through meditation.*

When we bring to full consciousness the true state of our being, the divine presence, we radiate the infinite in its fullness. When we think we are only this separate person, the contraction of the ego veils the truth.

Who we think this person is consists of illusory concepts and mental conditioning. This is the way the Self hides from Itself. The Self is revealed when the mind becomes still and we experience directly the presence that enlivens this form. Then we know beyond any doubt the true nature of our identity. We are waves of the absolute in the ocean of bliss.

The true teacher is one who lives fully in the transcendent state all the time and has the power to awaken others to this unlimited consciousness. Consider the inductance coil; the signal on one coil is transmitted by inductance to an adjacent coil. The signal is transmitted without distortion only if there is not already some signal on the second coil. Similarly, the full state is received by the student only if the student is free of interference and resistance. One can maintain this state by constant remembrance and choosing authenticity of perfection every moment.

In this Yoga of Discrimination, one discriminates the real from the illusory. The final discrimination is that only consciousness is real and everything else is unreal. From this it is realized that everything that is unreal is also consciousness.

Therefore, all is the one Self of existence, consciousness and bliss absolute.

That is what they say.

But what is meant by *real?* What is meant by *illusion?* There is something about the evidence of my own experience that tells me that this world is real. This inconsistency must be reconciled or yoga becomes just another mental trip.

Wisdom of the Yoga of Discrimination teaches that the only *real* is the immutable and eternal self-luminous consciousness. The *unreal* is whatever changes or is compounded and eventually disperses. So, *illusory,* in this context, means *ephemeral.* The enchantress *Maya* only calls one to the thralldom of the ephemeral, while the longing in our being call us to be reunited with the truth of our being; the immutable and eternal contentment of conscious awareness unfettered by the distraction of the mind.

Right use of intelligence is to reflect back upon itself and open the inner eye of Self-consciousness. Meditation is the treatment of choice for this infirmity of preoccupation with the ephemeral, which only leads to suffering.

~

Said a friend: *Oh, I get it! The game is to wake up before you die.* Nicely put.

It is the self-luminous consciousness of our own true nature seeing past the veil of the mind. It is our own divine Self awakening to the sacredness of all being. The catch is that the mind must be free of fantasy, must rest in stillness.

What went wrong? Why does the mind obsess over name and form? How come the species isn't naturally immersed in transcendence?

There is a seeking instinct that is common to all life: pseudopodia in amoeba; phototropism in plants; reptilia seeking movement and vibration, etc. This seeking is deeply rooted in the structures of our central nervous system, the brain stem or reptilian brain. It is inextricably linked with survival of the organism. The power of this instinct is demonstrated in our fascination for television and computers. Stuff on the screen moves, and we are captivated. Sport is about a moving target. When the ball stops, the game stops. And, it is not sporting to shoot a duck sitting still in the water.

As long as there are thoughts moving in the sensorium, we naturally follow them. Overcoming this tendency flies in the face of our deepest conditioning. This seeking instinct lives in the service of survival of the body and mind. However, we are neither the body nor the mind. Therefore this flight of fantasy only keeps us asleep to the bliss of being.

It is common for most people to strive to fill up their physical lives with attachment to possessions; to fill up their mental lives with attachment and aversion to ideals, concepts and beliefs; to fill up their emotional lives with attachment and aversion to personal relationships and righteous causes.

The great sadness is that all of this stuff is ephemeral, just a passing distraction, only the narcotic of craving and ignorance. This filling up of one's ego with the stuff of the world is precisely what weaves the shroud over knowledge of one's true identity.

To know the Self, to see clearly into the truth of being, is a process of emptying out all that is illusory. This is not just an exercise for the mind. One must disentangle one's life from the attachments, aversions, cravings, fear, and ignorance. Let it go. Wrench free from the quicksand of *Maya*. Turn the striving toward emptiness. Crave the emptiness. Embody the emptiness.

Then, in the stillness of meditation, look within and behold the self-luminous vastness of rapture. This is liberation. This is enlightenment. This is finding the Self by losing the self. This is becoming the divine presence.

Spiritual death is attained through desire for the ephemeral. Immortality is attained through awakening to the inner consciousness of the immutable and eternal state of unfettered awareness.

Immortality is when there is no more death. So how can there be immortality when we all die some day? First, we need to know what dies and what doesn't. The body dies. That is for sure. We have all seen dead bodies. The mind dies. To understand this better, we need to know that the mind has three constituent aspects: *manas, buddhi,* and *ahamkara. Manas* is the recording faculty that receives impressions gathered by the senses from the outside world. *Buddhi* is the discriminative faculty that classifies these impressions and reacts to them. *Ahamkara* is the ego that maintains the sense of individuality. When the body dies, these faculties no longer function, so the mind naturally expires with the body.

What is left?

A person has four bodies: gross, subtle, causal, and supra-causal. The gross body is the physical form. The subtle body is the carrier of karmic impressions as the *atman* migrates through successive incarnations. The causal body is the *pranic* force within the subtle body and is untouched by *karma.* The supra-causal body is the free and formless universal consciousness: immutable and immortal. As long as we think we are the physical body, we will die; then return to take another body because of our attachment to, and focus on, the form. When we turn within and discover the knower of the mind, we awaken to that which continues unaffected when the form falls away. To become established in the consciousness of the light of being behind the mind is to make the leap into immortality. That is when there is no more death.

Much has been said about the final state, but little about the method. There are many ways, but the goal is always the same. I personally prefer the most direct path with the least amount of glamour and obfuscation. Most important is having a teacher who is established in the state one wants to attain. From there, the most reliable tactics are to meditate, chant the Name, surrender, and attract the grace of the master.

Sanskrit is a revealed language. The ancient sages who gave us this powerful language would meditate upon certain phenomena until its noumena would reveal itself in a sound form that is the vibratory analogue of its essential nature: its true name. So, as one meditates upon a Sanskrit word, the phenomenon is translated from its noumenal vibration and is imprinted into the meditator. As a practical matter, this is how yogic powers are attained. Once the true name of the power is known, all that remains is to chant the name and the power manifests. Of course, in the mystical traditions, the main practice is to chant and meditate upon the Sanskrit names of nameless formless to drink in the divine essence. This works.

Surrender: what method can be used to surrender to the sweet equanimity of the divine absolute? It works exactly the same as surrendering to sleep. Be perfectly still and it will absorb you into itself. Perfect stillness of the body takes practice. Perfect stillness of the mind takes dedication. So, what is it that is surrendered? It is the sense of separate identity: the ego.

Attracting the grace of the master comes through surrender to the master, practicing the teachings of an enlightened being. Stilling the mind touches the source of grace.

The practices and restraints given in yoga and mysticism are for the purpose of conditioning the aspirant to bring to consciousness the nature of one's spirit-self. When the conscious soul leaves the limitation of the physical body, it is presented with a situation that is a critical turning point. Will the soul return to take another body on the plane of suffering because of its conditioning and attachment to the physical realm? Or, will it merge into the universal rapture of being from whence it emerged for the purpose of knowing itself?

The beacon of the Self broadcasts on a number of different frequencies: light, sound, bliss, sensory tranquility, love, pervasiveness, intelligence, awareness, and the *spanda* of being.

Practicing these attunements while still in the body builds familiarity and momentum to continue forward when the body falls away. The experience that greets the Self is so awesome that, unless it is already accustomed to the light and power, its tendency is to turn away to the familiarity of the darkness. One knows a great being not by how he lives, but by *how he dies*.

Sri Yukteswar defines a *Siddha* as one who is established in that steady state, such that he is beyond the influence of the *matrika shakti* of ideas or concepts. Our task is indeed to attain the steady state beyond the sway of the mind. We make the choice now whether we will return to the limitation and suffering; for beyond this plane, the mind will not be there to help us figure things out. We have to already be where we are going. Otherwise, we do it all over again.

I hope it is obvious that the best guidance on this path is a living master who is fully established in the final state. With only a few on the planet, it is rare indeed to have the grace to be chosen by one and accept the challenge to become liberated while still in the body. It is a challenge fulfilled through turning inward and knowing the divine Self in the inner light, the inner sound, awareness of pure being, effulgence of peace, bliss and love, and expanding into the universal power of conscious awareness.

Of course, if one does not have even the slightest longing for liberation, all of the above is merely psychobabble.

All of yoga is preparation for the last moment before — and the first moment after— leaving the body. Become the impassive witness. Meet adversity with indifference. Every experience is taking the *darshan* of the Self. The heart of austerity is about simplicity — not about mortification.

Awakening into immortality emerges from the full awareness of being in which the attention is not distracted by the dance of the senses or impressions from the mind. To attain the immortal state while still in the body requires the finest discrimination and uncompromising effort to hold the *khechari mudra.* The pure state of *khechari* is in the experience that one's identity is but movement in the vastness of consciousness. This is what remains when the noise of the body and mind is stilled; this is what continues when the *prana* abandons the form; this is the immortal, or true Self. All else is ephemeral, therefore not real. This immortal presence longs to be remembered through the veil of illusion and is present in its fullness every moment. All that is required is to lose interest in the psychodrama, detach from the senses, and surrender to the source of grace. *Grace* is one of those long-standing undefined mysteries first encountered in childhood. Everybody I asked told me what they thought grace was, but I could tell that they really didn't know. Webster's Dictionary authoritatively tells us that *grace* is divine assistance with sanctification; and Roget's says that *sanctity* is something like purity. This is okay, but I want something that touches my heart with truth.

Naturally, we get everything we ask for; so, this week, in a letter from an enlightened being, I am told that, *Grace is that natural force which causes the experience of merging.* Well, now I get it. Of course. It is all becoming clear.

For the first time, I understand what is meant by the saying, *The purpose of the guru is to dispense grace.* And, in the guru's own words, *The thought-free state is the source of grace.* Ahh, a great mystery solved.

But again, it is one thing for the mind to become dis-impaled from the prong of an enigma, and quite another to have the experience.

It is subtle indeed to actually perceive that natural force that causes the experience of merging. It absolutely requires that the clamor of the senses be stilled or ignored — this includes the caroming of the mind. Once in the still state, one is astonished by how noisy this earthly vehicle is, and how attentive one must be to entice substance from the workings of grace. When the longing is great, then the Force is strong. Grace quickens the reunion of the sleeper with the awakened who were never separate, but only dreaming.

~

*gate gate paragate parasamgate bodhi svaha*

This ancient Buddhist chant may best be translated as:

*Gone, gone, utterly gone, gone without recall. O freedom!*

. . . *gone without recall? Gone beyond remembering ever having been? O freedom!* It is true. Meditation on the purity of our ultimate nature leads us inexorably to the most subtle realm of being. Once one is established in the steady state of joyous tranquility, one merges spontaneously into the causal state where there is no one else who might have been. What grace to have been shown this experience.

We are as droplets of ocean spray who imagine we have been flung into separation from the rapture. The shock of estrangement projects an intense longing to remerge with the one we are the same as.

The fear of loneliness sends us into a frenzy of grasping for one who will embrace us with endless bliss, one into whom we can merge and forget the unbearable emptiness.

We know we have this merging urging, but what we are confused about is what will bring fulfillment and contentment.

As long as we pursue satisfaction in the realm of the ephemeral, then the embrace will bear the kiss of separation, and we will be no closer to resolving our most fundamental torment: the angst in the mind.

If, however, we turn within and retrace the forgotten path to the immortal light of being, then all our longing is dissolved in the joy of remembrance. We merge into the presence of the beloved when the caprice of the mind comes to rest.

The sublime transcendence of the inner hush commutes distraction into nectar and every vibration becomes a reflection of the divine *spanda*.

There is a secret place in my heart where just the beloved dwells. I enter there only in perfect stillness, but as I enter there, I cease to be. There is a threshold where separateness coalesces into the absolute; the particular sublimates into vastness; contraction releases into love and "I" merge into the beloved.

~

*Dharma* is another one of those concepts seemingly cloaked in mystery. Perhaps it is because there have been so many different translations of that Sanskrit word, such as: work, destiny, life purpose, right action, etc. An illumined one gives us a hint in saying that *climbing a mountain may seem impossible, but, in taking the next step, dharma is fulfilled.*

The Mahabharata tells us that a person's *dharma* is supported by eight qualities: austerity, charity, study, sacrifice, truthfulness, forgiveness, compassion, and contentment. Righteousness is sustained through these noble virtues. One's dharmic path is always clear in the light of righteousness.

Still, we must remember that beyond righteous *dharma* is liberation. The Chandogya Upanishad says that: *the lives of those who follow the eight virtues are blest, [. . .] but he who is firmly established in the knowledge of Brahman achieves immortality.*

Everyone is in orbit around some thing, some one, some notion, or some experience. If the object of the primary orbit is a manifestation of the ephemeral realm, then one remains arrested in the *perpetuum mobile* of death and *karma*. Once, however, the attention becomes fixed on the supreme inner stillness, one finally merges into the radiance of eternal rapture, free at last from the captivity of forgetfulness and suffering.

When the cultural window dressing is set aside, and we cut through the mystical metaphor, the so called *spiritual path* leads us to re-experience the personal equipoise that was forgotten when the senses turned toward the stimulation of the ephemeral world.

Unless our memory of the boundless rapture is especially strong, or we find a perfected master to teach us, then we may never, in this incarnation, remember to remember. Life becomes wishful pursuit of short-lived pleasure, and desperate grasping for money, possession, and relationships to distract us from the emptiness. In the end, however, only one thing works ... to rediscover the fullness of perpetual love and joy of our true nature that was always here all along.

~

All this talk about merging.... What is it, really? Certainly it's a fine concept, even a sublime concept. But let's get real; exactly what is the *experience* of merging about?

In the Vedic tradition there is a Sanskrit invocation that goes something like this:

> *Om.*
> *Pure consciousness* (That) *is full and perfect;*
> *the manifest universe* (This) *is full and perfect.*
> *From perfect consciousness springs the perfection of the*
> *ephemeral world of name and form.*
> *When* _this_ *fullness merges in that fullness, all that*
> *remains is fullness.*
> *Om. Shanti. Shanti. Shanti.*

The great eighth century saint, Shankaracharya, notes here that the term "merges" refers to the realization that the universe is *Brahman*. We know that this manifest universe originated in and contracted from the supreme absolute pure consciousness, and, in fact, still is that. Therefore, we come to experience our phenomenal world as divine. This is like the sage who, upon being approached by someone, says, *Ah Shiva, you have come to me in this form.* This is merging.

Remember grace... *that natural force which causes the experience of merging?* As we mature spiritually, through the power of will, we begin to see the divine in each other. Grace removes the obstacles to experiencing this world as divine.

~

Long ago and far, far away, the sage Vasishta, giving instruction to his pupil, the avatar Rama, tells him the story of the awakening of King Janaka. At the moment of revelation the great king reflected to himself:

"O unsteady mind, reach the state of equanimity, for then you will experience peace, bliss and truth. Give up all hopes and expectations, and freed from the wish to seek or to abandon, roam about freely. Do not let the apparent merits and demerits of this world-appearance disturb your equanimity."

Now, the case of Rama is very interesting. Everyone knew that Rama was a divine incarnation—except Rama himself. It was only after being instructed by the sage Vasishta that he learned his true identity.

We too are Rama. Steeped in ignorance, we only learn of our true nature after being instructed by the sage. The Consciousness itself is revealed as our innermost being.

Great longing, uncompromising discipline in doing the practices every day, right understanding that the true guru is the state; study of the scriptures, lifetimes of merit, and the grace of a living master makes liberation in this lifetime possible. Hey, and this is fun too — great joy in all of it. There is nothing in the ephemeral world that delivers eternal unconditional love.

The guru is transparent to the divine Self within. She shows us our highest potential. How can we not surrender utterly to that true love that lives within, as us?

For us to attain that full radiance of seamless unbounded love we must share her state deeply. The guru's state is calm and clear (*nirvikalpa*). A Siddha is simultaneously aware of the inner focus (*shunyavidya*) as well as outer events. It takes practice but this state is attainable by each of us. There are even instructions provided in the Vijnanabhairava.

This yoga is so practical. It is also concise, clear, and verifiable in experience. That is what I like about it — second best. First best I like the sweetness it brings to life and the everpresent joy of being.

# Perspectives East and West

## Conscious Substratum

Existence comes in two flavors: the changing, and the unchanging. The changing is defined as that which is created from something else. Nature is the changing. It is built up from hydrogen from the birth of the universe. Hydrogen fuses to create other elements, which make up all objects of nature.

Everything that exists was either created from something else, or has always existed. Consciousness is not created from something else, so has always existed. Even our universe of changing space-time is a special case within the existence of consciousness.

The unchanging is universal consciousness, and is the substratum of all being. Some objects in nature are asleep to consciousness, and others are awake and self-aware. Consciousness is the knower; nature is the known. Consciousness cannot be an object of awareness because it is the watcher; and there is no watcher of the watcher.

Only a few will discover the inner stillness, where consciousness is Self-aware. It is the mind that is in the way of awakening to transcendent consciousness. Most are continuously infatuated with the entertainment of personal drama; only a few will touch the stillness. Fewer still, will become the stillness.

What is the mind and where did it come from? Consciousness becomes the mind, contracted by objects in the appearance. When consciousness takes the form of the mind, consciousness cannot be aware of itself. Only the mind suffers, and we find pristine happiness in the stillness. *Sadhana* is redirecting the focus of consciousness to the stillness of just being. Once we become established in this stillness, we are finished.

## Principles of Yoga Philosophy
### 1. Consciousness and the mind are different.
Consciousness is the witness of the the mind. The mind is local to the brain but consciousness is non-local. When the brain dies, the mind dies; but consciousness, the universal field, remains. The mind is a complex instrument of perception that includes ego, memory and rationality. In the intimate relationship between consciousness and the mind, consciousness is the perceiver, the mind is the instrument of perceiving. Importantly, consciousness can know the mind but the mind cannot know consciousness.

To understand this better we need to know that the mind has three constituent aspects: memory (*manas*), intellect (*buddhi*), and ego (*ahamkara*). *Manas* is the recording faculty that receives impressions gathered by the senses from the outside world. *Buddhi* is the discriminative faculty that classifies these impressions and reacts to them. *Ahamkara* is the ego that maintains the sense of individuality. When the body dies these faculties no longer function so the mind naturally expires with the body. When we turn within and discover the knower of the mind, we awaken to that which continues unaffected when the form falls away. To become established in the consciousness of the light of being behind the mind is to make the leap into immortality. That is when there is no more death.

### 2. The causes of suffering are:
a) Attachment and aversion
b) Concern for gain and loss.

It is common for most people to strive to fill up their physical life with attachment to possessions; to fill up their mental life with attachment and aversion to ideals, concepts and beliefs; to fill up their emotional life with attachment and aversion to personal relationships and righteous causes.

The great sadness is that all of this stuff is ephemeral, just a passing distraction, only the narcotic of craving and ignorance. This filling up of one's ego with the stuff of the world is precisely what weaves the shroud over knowledge of one's true identity.

To know the Self, to see clearly into the truth of being, is a process of emptying out all that is illusory. This is not just an exercise for the mind. One must disentangle one's life from the attachments, aversions, cravings and ignorance.

A Sufi master once wrote: *You get two things in life; that which you love and that which you hate.* Dissolution of ego and liberation from attachment and avoidance brings to an end all *karma* associated with things you love and things you hate.

Basically, liberation is awakening from the accumulated ignorance that comes with living in the world, believing that we're imperfect, having attachments and aversions, thinking that anything is important, and feeling that we are separate beings.

*Jnana yoga* discriminates the real from the illusory and brings one to the awareness of the blissful and pure inner Self. When desire and attachment have been overcome and the mind rests in utter serenity, when the ego-sense dissolves into absolute consciousness, then one is liberated from the wheel of death and rebirth. If we never relinquish our identity with, and attachment to the body and other ephemeral stuff, we will follow that attachment back into another body for yet another round on the karmic wheel.

Our characteristic beliefs, expectations and interests are created from attachment, aversion, compulsions, identification, addiction and inhibition. These are the six deadly sins. Become established in the joyous tranquility of the inner Self so that when the body suddenly drops away we will not be distracted by attachments to the world. In this way the Soul will complete its journey home. All of yoga is preparation for the last moment before, and the first moment after, leaving the body. So it appears that destiny is partly ordained by karma and partly determined by the desires of our mind. All the more reason to meditate and purify our minds of idle attachments and aversions to focus on attainments that will bring us liberation for eternity rather than pleasure for the moment.

*Know the Self*

The mind is not different from the thoughts it thinks. Thoughts arise from past impressions. The ego has the power to sequence the thoughts so that they make sense to the intellect. Streams of thought in the waking state have coherency because of the sequencer, the ego. Thought streams from past impressions in the dream state lack coherency because of the absence of the sequencer.

Beginning meditation, stillness of *prana* brings stillness to the mind. In the end, stilling the mind bring stillness to *prana*.

In the stillness of meditation, the mind is restrained, reveling in the love that spontaneously shines from the heart. This sweetness of peace and bliss comes from our own true inner Self to ourself. The mind could feel guilty about this and think it is selfish and narcissistic, but the mind is wrong. Stilling the mind is opening the heart. Go deep into the stillness and let the Self shine your own love on you. It is your true nature; it is who you really are.

In the stillness of meditation we experience pure awareness of just being. In this awareness of just being is the peaceful presence that is our true inner Self. It is like looking into the eyes of another and seeing yourself looking back at you. Try this!

Who am I? Who are you? Who are we? Am I the mind? Am I the body? The body is just dirt and water. The mind is totally imaginary. The Self that is alive is the conscious indweller. And the local indweller is not different than Universal Consciousness. Within is the infinite, eternal, and unchanging Self. We cannot know or experience that as long as the mind is in the way. Meditate, still the mind; know the Self.

## Be Present

Wake up from the dream of the mind. Sit quietly every day and touch the stillness; you will get everything in this practice.

The past and future are completely illusory, true reality is only in the present now. Learn to live in a world where there is no past or future. Simply be present in the boundaryless bliss of now. Here we merge into the eternal unity of consciousness, the Self.

Consciousness is the essence of sentiency.

## Why Stillness?

The inner stillness is always happy and content.

In this stillness is a peacefulness that can never be disturbed.

In this stillness is the love that will never leave you.

This stillness brings the wisdom that surpasses all knowledge.

This stillness is the aliveness that remains when the body falls away.

## Stages of Spiritual Sadhana

1. **Purification**
2. **Transmission**
3. **Transcendent Steady State**

The beginning of spiritual sadhana is purification of the mind through meditation discipline and taking the meditative state out into the world, as much as possible.

Transmission is in two phases. The outer phase is learning, through study and practice, the exoteric meaning of the transcendent state. The inner phase is learning through direct knowing, the fullness of the emptiness.

Transcendence is being established in the inner stillness. living your life from the place of the peaceful presence.

## The Problem
**You want something you don't have.**
**You have something you don't want.**
**You want something to be other than it is.**
**You want someone to be different than they are.**

There appear to be four problems, but there is only one problem—the mind. The solution to the problem is to become the watcher of the mind; then lose interest in the drama.

In the stillness, the impartial witness transcends the suffering of the mind and attains freedom.

## Our Sadhana
It's quite simple really, we are already enlightened and perfect;
only the mind is in the way of realization.
Our *sadhana* is the practices that bring the mind to stillness: meditation, kirtan, reverence, and gratitude.

## Surrender
Surrender is a word that is not usually heard in polite company. In normal usage it infers defeat, humiliation, and capitulation in combat. Antithetically, on the spiritual path, surrender is essential to attain the goal of liberation. In the beginning one surrenders to the teachings, to the will, and to the grace of the master. This leads ultimately to inner surrender to the thought free state that opens one fully to divine inspiration, perpetual joy, and perfect serenity.

The Sufis call this "fana" which is usually translated as annihilation. The traditional progression is fana-fi-sheikh, fana-fi-pir, and fana-fi-Allah, or progressive annihilation into the teacher, the master, and the Absolute.

What has to be surrendered is the pride of ego and the sense of separation. It is a gradual process but has to start somewhere. The student must decide at some point that he or she needs help from a higher source, that what he has figured out to do doesn't work.

In February of 1980 upon returning from India, I learned that my grant funded position was not renewed. All my savings had gone for the trip, and the house I had just bought was going to require mortgage payments. All my efforts to find employment failed and I was in deep despair. I needed help. On my knees with face to the floor I prayed: If there is anyone up there who knows or cares, I need you now, I can't do this on my own. In that very instant, a perfectly composed and serene Indian woman in sari and shawl appeared before my eyes and gazed at me intently for a long time. She said nothing, but by the intensity of her eyes I felt that she looked into my very soul.

It is as if the guru had waited for my moment of surrender to appear. When they say that the master appears when the student is ready, here, ready means surrendered. The curious thing about this incident is that it wasn't until two years later that she was initiated as the successor to the Siddha lineage by her guru. The guru is so mysterious.

Subsequent to the inner surrender is the welcoming of every experience in life, pleasurable as well as painful. In this surrender to life as it is, one honors karma and appreciates the wisdom of the *shakti* in bringing us what is right for the moment. The mind becomes free of resistance and avoidance and becomes liberated from desire and expectations. The ego thereby dissolves leaving only the divine presence to enjoy the play.

A Sufi master once wrote: *You get two things in life—that which you love and that which you hate.* Dissolution of ego, and liberation from attachment and avoidance, brings to an end all karma associated with things you love and things you hate. We sentenced ourselves to this incarnation to finish with what we loved and hated in previous incarnations. Seeds of karma are sewn out of strong opinions, so one of the things we are here to finish with is our opinions.

We have come back to finish with many things. All our significant relationships are hanging there, waiting to be finished. Don't be afraid just to let go. Even new relationships come to us in order to be released. Honor the process, play it out, and let it go. Even our present physical circumstances have manifested out of previous desires. Continuing to desire a particular circumstance will bring us back to have it again.

We must take inventory of what our predominant focus of attention is on, and understand the profundity of consequence of this focus. If there is even the slightest clutching on to things of the ephemeral realm, as we merge into the beyond, then around we go again. Letting go of everything every moment frees us in the present and frees us in eternity.

Disentangling from the world does not have to be a painful process. It does not require severe austerity or penance. It is not like pulling out your own teeth or hacking off your leg. Once the inner wellspring of love is tasted, we see that everything we ever craved in the world flows abundantly from within. There is a natural turning to face the source of perpetual sweetness of serenity. In this turning toward the light, there is a pliant relenting of our grip on things and relationships that once held us in thrall. As we drink in the nectar of the soul, we gradually forget the importance of our attachments. They release us, as we embrace the love and wisdom of our own inner Self.

The murmur of the inner love is faint in the face of the presiding ego with its desires and fears. For the whisper to become a rush of rapture, the ego has to go. This is a problem, since the ego resists annihilation rather vigorously. The power of this apparition is great. Having been created out of the power of the Absolute to hide from Itself, the ego mimics the powers of *iccha, jnana* and *kriya shakti*; or will, knowledge and action. Even though the illusory ego possesses these powers in limited form, they are still powers to be reckoned with. Theoretically, perhaps, through the ego's power of knowledge, it could understand that it gets in the way of bliss and use its *shaktis* of *iccha* and *kriya* to dissolve itself— it just doesn't work out that way. So, what to do?

The divine power to hide gives us the ego. Fortunately the Self has the power to reveal itself, also called the power of grace. This power resides with a true guru. The guru, dispensing grace, reveals to us our divine nature. She frees us not by bashing the ego into submission but by giving us the experience of the Self through *shaktipat* and by giving us practices to attune us to the nectarian presence of our unbounded being.

Gradually over time, the ego fades from prominence due to lack of interest. The ego is seen for what it is, an imaginary shell of empty constructs that requires constant feeding and is never satisfied. It thinks it is somebody leading an interesting and important existence, but there is no such person. It thinks there is knowledge to be gained and attainments to strive for, but the only truth is illumined through surrender.

Because of the nagging childhood quest to know the truth, I took a fair amount of philosophy coursework to find the truth about the nature of reality. It was one of my greatest college disappointments that the study of philosophy was limited to rational epistemologies. Philosophy was not about the nature of reality, but it was about ways of knowing, or perspectives on knowledge. They were little more than various elaborations on Plato's cave allegory.

What good fortune it is to have contact with an order of monks whose work is to give the experience of the ultimate reality as well as to teach the rational philosophy of a meta-rational (transcendental) epistemology.

In the philosophical or scriptural authority of this order of monks, the Ultimate Reality is called *Paramashiva*. This fundamental ground-state of being is non-relational consciousness, the Supreme Self surveying Itself, the subject void of object. It is also known as *prakasha-vimarshamaya*. This Sanskrit name implies two aspects of the Ultimate Reality: 1) *Prakasha*: the principle of self-revelation or illumination by which everything is hknown, and 2) *Vimarsha*: the power of consciousness to know Itself. Maya is the power of *Vimarsha* that differentiates the knower from the known.

*Prakasha* is the experiencing principle and *Vimarsha* is the projecting principle. The kinetic aspect is the seed of all emanations and is responsible for the manifestation, maintenance and reabsorption of the universe. This dynamic mirror of the splendor of Shiva is called Shakti. Her powers are will, knowledge, and action. She is the first throb of distinction and brings immanence to the transcendental undifferentiated Paramashiva.

This dance of emerging and re-merging is experienced in meditation. When the yogi is in the steady thought-free state, pure consciousness observes itself by its own illumination; the universe of differentiation exists only as potential in the unmanifest. When a thought arises in the mind (thought is the mind), a universe of illusory non-Self has been created. When consciousness returns to perfect tranquillity, the display of imagination resorbs back into the transcendent undifferentiated consciousness.

On a different scale, the Self differentiates when the *jiva* (empirical self) takes birth for another karmic incarnation. On a grand scale, the entire universe of all manifestation becomes abstract potential when *Shakti* withdraws her powers and merges once again into Paramashiva.

It is interesting to note that a principal point of difference between Vedanta and Kashmir Shaivism is that Kashmir Shaivism teaches that the Ultimate Reality possesses, in the unmanifest, the dynamic power to project the latent universe. Vedanta teaches that the Ultimate Reality is void of even the potential of activity. Vedanta seems to be unclear about the origin of *Maya Shakti*.

This difference also helps to explain that the lineage of monks who teach Kashmir Shaivism is a shaktipat lineage. They command the power of consciousness to illumine the seeker after truth. Experiencing the transmission of shakti renders the scriptures of Kashmir Shaivism self-evident. Hence, true knowledge is revealed to the mind, and transcendence reveals pure consciousness observing itself. All this is verifiable in experience, therefore it is the truth beyond any opinion, belief, inference, or theory.

All this discussion of truth is, of course, within the framework that anything that can be thought, written or inferred is not it. The truth of the Ultimate Reality is only in the immutable, eternal, unchanging Absolute. We become the Absolute through the opening of the heart.

Okay, so what does it mean to open the heart? My general impression has been that we know with the mind and feel in the heart; that the heart center is the core of emotional content. If this is the case, then what is the connection between emotions and the divine unmanifest?

The Sanskrit word "*hrdaya*" in its literal sense means heart. However, in its esoteric, mystical, or spiritual usage, it means the center of pure consciousness, or the Self. As a scholar of Tantra Yoga once wrote: *As the heart opens, there is a sense of merging.*

One merges into objectless awareness of being. This is the opening of the heart. Over time, through intention, one becomes established in this steady state of contented perfection.

As for the task of living in the world while immersed in the steady state of unflappable tranquillity, one draws intelligence and guidance from the inspiration of direct knowing. The obstacle of mental concern no longer obscures the wisdom of intuition. Whatever comes is welcomed; whatever goes is released.

The inspiration that we tap into as we turn inward toward the source of happiness is the everflowing fountain of infinite joy, boundless freedom, and perfect contentment. Even though the opening of the mystical heart does not promise romance, it gradually immerses us in the love we have longed for since the soul took form. As long as we are focused on the inner flow of inspiration, we are complete in the remembrance of our true Self. When we are distracted by ephemeral temptation, we forget temporarily the perfection of just being.

If there is anything worth striving for, it is to hold this awareness of steady wisdom. The Shiva Sutras say that the highest use of will is to remain in the highest state. A great contemporary saint teaches that to attain the highest we must love our own soul completely.

So how do we love our soul completely? For me, at least, a great love for the soul didn't just appear when I had the desire to attain the highest. Our usual model for love is the romantic feelings of caring and the wish to be with the beloved as much as possible. There is much new learning involved as we create a love relationship with our own Self. As in any relationship it begins with desire for there to be a relationship; an attraction. Then the relationship is nurtured by spending time together. In this case, meditation is the beginning of being alone together to get acquainted. The mantra is used to purify the mind and clear a space to share intimate moments of being merged in each other. We find that the soul is a little shy and doesn't always rush to meet us, so we must be patient as well as persistent to gain the full trust of the beloved.

As we spend more and more time together, we become more familiar with the nature of the one we have waited so long to embrace. Great longing and constant remembrance turns our attention to feeling the constant presence of the sweet love that we know will be ours forever. There are times when we just cannot bear the separation and pine for moments alone, just the one of us.

We feel, more and more, the love of the Self with us constantly. We experience the radiance of the divine presence that enlivens our very being. Finally, we merge into the bliss of the eternal source of all manifestation. No more you and me. Separation is forgotten. Only love.

In the inevitable turning of the wheel, the illumined inner eye of compassion turns to peer out into the plane of the manifest. The Self sees into other eyes of Itself and remembers the sublime unity of pure awareness. We also observe the illusory drama of ego and the workings of karma. With the eye of compassion, we watch the dance of action and reaction, understanding that the sleeping have only their conditioning to show us. But we see only the beloved; waiting.

Seeing only the Self in each other transforms our life and opens us to our divine qualities of loving dispassion, inner tranquillity, and inspired wisdom. This is, however, a gradual process, and it is helpful to remember that, in the beginning, bliss is only the absence of suffering. As the light of the Self gradually emerges into conscious awareness through persistent meditation, we sink into the familiarity of the divine presence.

Meditation is only one of three primary strategies to know the Self and attain the highest state. A great Indian saint says emphatically that it is a law that if you meditate and chant and love the guru, you will attain liberation. Each of these strategies are complete yogas in themselves, and each ultimately leads to liberation — but why not practice all three simultaneously? These practices are in no way mutually exclusive, in fact they are complimentary and enhance each other synergistically.

An insightful monk in the Saraswati Order told me that, meditation is to still the mind; chanting is to open the heart. In its most sublime form, chanting is the singing of divine names to entreat the Self to manifest the divine presence within us. It is customary to chant the name in its Sanskrit form. Powerful

Sanskrit mantras have been given to us by meditation masters and are considered to be alive with the power of consciousness. One reason that this practice has persisted for so many thousands of years is that it works.

Stilling the mind through meditation brings to the foreground the highest state of consciousness. Chanting the name opens the heart to the bliss of the Self. The third prescription, loving the guru, evokes the grace to merge into the Universal Absolute.

To the uninitiated, loving the guru might be met with skepticism. So we should know who the guru is. The true guru is our own inner Self. The form of the outer guru is one who is perfectly clear and transparent to the state, the love, and the power of the divine Absolute. We express unabashed gratitude to the guru for showing us ourselves. Loving the guru is not different than loving our own soul completely. To experience this is to understand how loving the guru is a complete yoga, and how it is harmonious with meditation and chanting, and how it all leads to liberation.

Ah, liberation. But liberation from what? Basically, liberation is awakening from the accumulated ignorance that comes with living in the world, believing that we're imperfect, having attachments, aversions, and fears; thinking that anything is important, and feeling that we are separate beings. Ignorance must be an utterly fascinating subject as there is a great deal written about it. So, to get right to the root of the most fundamental ignorance, consider the teaching in the Shiva Sutras that the primary ignorance is forgetting that our true identity is pure consciousness. Naturally, when we remember who we are, we become liberated. Easier said than done.

It gets more complicated and the muck of ignorance gets deeper. It is not enough that the power of illusion causes us to forget the bliss of heaven; this cleavage of perspective causes the bereft Soul to take form in the physical plane and experience separation. As a consequence of committing willful actions out of ignorance, karma is created that entrains the individual soul to innumerable lifetimes of suffering.

There's more.

Yet even a thicker plot of stupefaction arises in the mind in the form of constructs, i.e., thoughts and feelings. It is perhaps the power of words that is the most terrible enemy of divine light. This frivolous prattle of inanity holds us prisoner lifetime after lifetime. One is mired in the dark pit of bondage not having a clue about how to find happiness. Everything one craves only brings more suffering. Satisfaction is short lived, and emptiness grows as possessions and self-importance pile up. Despair increases, and drugs, sex, and rock 'n roll don't fill up the holes any more.

Then one day, inexplicably, a sudden flash of divine consciousness emerges from within, perhaps by the will of a Siddha Master. The pilgrim tastes the indelible nectar of truth. The sweetness lingers, the light shines, the power expands, the love emerges, and serenity pervades the conscious awareness of the one who longs for union with the beloved.

This little drama of the power of the Self to hide from Itself, and then reveal Itself, is illuminated in the Shiva Sutras. Commentary on the sutras explains that the Self exists as pure awareness of being in unmanifest absolute unity. That is, until the veil of *anava mala* obscures the transcendence of Self-knowledge and also gives rise to *mayiya mala* and *karma mala*. In this way the power of the Absolute to create the illusion of separation is manifest. *Anava mala* is the first forgetfulness. *Mayiya mala* is the sense of differentiation. We experience this in the thought that I am this body and my Self is different from your Self. *Karma mala* empowers the empirical person to create karma due to actions performed under the bondage of *mayiya mala*. The final corruption arises from *matrika shakti*: the power of thought to get completely in the way of perceiving the highest state that exists all the time, just behind the mind. (Shiva Sutras, Jaideva Singh ed., Sutra #2 pp. 16 - 21. Motilal Barnisidass. Delhi, India, 1979)

Thus we have the totally ignorant person stumbling around frightened and semi-crazed through a fog of nearly irredeemable delusion. Or, we could see this as a fully enlightened being playing at the sport of forgetfulness until the descent of grace liberates the soul into the rapture of eternity.

In either case, all that is really happening is the dance of light and shadow, the drama of knowledge and ignorance. As such, it is a thoroughly eastern view of things. It is interesting to compare this paradigm with the western religious view of how things seem to be.

For the sake of brevity we will consider only the fundamental dichotomies of each system. In the east, the fundamental dichotomy is knowledge and ignorance, i.e., knowledge of (actually, experience of) the eternal bliss of the supreme Absolute, and ignorance of same. In the west the fundamental dichotomy is good and evil. Good in the Judeo-Christian tradition generally means actions sanctioned by the ten commandments. Evil commonly arises from broken commandments and is attended by judgment and moral condemnation. This conduct ethic is our conscience from the cradle to the grave. Society is always pleased with us for being good persons, and doesn't everyone worry all their lives about the final judgment? Evil people are considered psychopaths and should be killed before they eat our children. I mean, isn't evil the most horrible and feared thing in the western culture?

There is moral condemnation in breaking the commandments, fear of condemnation in the final judgment and extreme condemnation for the insidiously evil. It's everywhere, it's everywhere.

Let us look again at the eastern fundamental dichotomy of knowledge and ignorance. Knowledge in this context means being Self-realized, enlightened, or established in the highest state. At the opposite end of the scale is ignorance, which basically means not enlightened yet. Ignorance only implies not being fully established in divine consciousness that leads to liberation. There is no condemnation in ignorance because it is just the normal state that most people are in as they go through this incarnation. Everyone knows that in this or some future incarnation that they will attain liberation, that is, full knowledge of the Self and liberation from the wheel of karma.

In the Hindu tradition a person goes through four stages in life: apprentice, householder, forest dweller, and sage. From this we see that the whole momentum of the culture is toward a life of awareness of one's true nature. Isn't it remarkable that there is much less condemnation in the religious and social fabric of this eastern culture? There is no hell. The worst possible thing that can happen is that an ignorant person will be reborn again in the physical plane and be ignorant again.

Acceptance of the human condition is not due to the lack of a conduct ethic. A very specific guideline of observances and restraints are codified in the Yoga Sutras of Patanjali. The observances (niyamas) are purification, contentment, scriptural study and mantra repetition, austerity, and devotion. The restraints are non-injury, truthfulness, non-stealing, continence, and non-attachment. (Yoga Sutras: The Means to Liberation, Dennis Hill, Trafford Publishing, 2007. Book II, sutras 29 - 42, pp. 62-70.)

This code of virtues is not intended so much as crowd control, but as a way to attain nobility of character and peace of mind. In the final analysis we find that practicing the observances and restraints bring us serenity and removes the obstacles to deeper and deeper experience of the Self. It's true; see for yourself that neglecting even a single one of the yamas or niyamas results in disturbance of the mind and nagging interruption of meditation.

Unveiling the mystery of the Self is very simple, really. We recognize two aspects of the Divine. One is the individual soul (Atma) and the other, the universal Self (Brahman). The Self is the light, power and intelligence of the Divine that enlivens and shines through our individual being. Brahman, the universal, is the source of the Divine light, power and intelligence that we call the Self.

We can think of *Atma* as a ray of the Self, or a limited aspect of the unlimited universal Absolute. In any case, the individual is not essentially different from the universal Absolute, right? We are the local address of the immutable, eternal, unchanging Absolute.

As we mature out of our anthropomorphic vision of God as the ethereal patriarch sitting in judgment over his creation, something not so wonderful happens. God becomes abstract; nothing to hold on to.

All is not lost, however. In the west there is Jesus who was a real person and acts as the representative or embodiment of God for all practical purposes. This is good in that it offers a higher power to believe in, community for mutual identity and support, the affirmation of ritual, the promise that we are loved in spite of our sins, and if we don't screw up too badly, we might get to heaven. For the most part, this is satisfactory.

If this is not satisfactory, it may mean one of two things. Either the whole thing seems delusional and it's easier not to believe any of it, or it's not enough and we want more and deeper. If we want more and deeper, it means going for the experience of the Self beyond the available knowledge about the divine. To have this experience, we must trace the thread of Selfhood back from the divine manifestation of creation through the individual to universal consciousness. Not an easy task.

In the book of Romans, Paul says that if you think you are the body you will die. The legacy of eternal life is gained by knowing oneself as Spirit.

So how do we do this?

Spiritual self-knowledge is awakened only by seeking the kingdom within through meditation. Bring the body into repose, forget the body, we are not the body, look inward. Bring the mind to repose, forget the mind, we are not the mind, look inward. The light, the power and the intelligence of the divine presence has been waiting for this moment of remembrance.

The Catholic Order of Monks of the Hezechast who historically lived in remote caves in North Africa practiced the discipline of silent meditation to remain in deep communion with the Absolute. Beyond this it is not doctrine anywhere else in the church. There are, of course, cloistered orders where individuals may practice the ecstatic thought-free state, and occasional mystics and saints. But elsewhere, it's a secret.

Because of meditation's occult reputation, it was overlooked in the Reformation of the 16th century. In the zeal of Martin Luther to be free from Catholic dogma, he pitched out the baby with the bathwater. As a result Protestants of today can't reach even a vestige of the mystical tradition that teaches meditation to open oneself to the full experience of the divine presence. Nothing is ultimately lost, however, and the aspirant who really wants it will find it.

The Vatican, years ago, published an Edict against the study or practice of yoga. It was explained that yoga might lead to physical cultism. At first Hatha Yoga teaches how to assume the correct poses; next, sustaining the *asanas* and *mudras* of the body is taught. After the body is taught to sustain stillness, the mind is taught to sustain stillness.

Stillness of mind is the posture of the finished yogi or yogini. This is called *khechari mudra*. Literally, *khechari* means movement in space. The most refined understanding of this *mudra* is where the yogi is merged in the consciousness that moves in all beings. This is mastery in meditation.

# Identity and Cosmology

Eight years ago I mused into my journal the following:

Recently I've begun to get an inkling of things yet to come. So far, meditation has been easy sitting in a dark silent room with eyes closed experiencing the fullness of pure consciousness beyond the seduction of the mind. That's nice, to be sure; peaceful, and even a happy time. But there is also meditation to practice out in the world. There is seeing beyond looking, listening beyond hearing, feeling beyond touching, knowing beyond thinking.

Unfocusing the mind amidst the word drama brings the light of wisdom, and indifference to the caprices of thought. How about unfocusing the sight, and indifference to the play on the screen? What realm of vision awaits this pilgrim around the next bend on the path?

This "realm of vision" that I knew would come, was described perfectly in a recent letter from an enlightened meditation teacher. He relates:

"Instead of seeing solid form, it is more like seeing dancing images from some invisible projector, seeing the light more than form. It's like meditating with our eyes open. As we go into meditation with open eyes, we take our focus off the usual forms that fascinate and entrance us. As we unfocus in this way, the world, as we usually know it, begins to disappear. We see through the world. We see through *maya*. It's like peering into the formless, into eternity; when we see through this world, we see the Self, Universal Consciousness."

In meditation we learn to see thoughts as bubbles of pure consciousness. In the pottery shop we see the bowls all as clay; similarly, in the world, we see the ephemeral forms as dancing images of light. We see through *maya* to behold the form of the formless. This is the realm of vision where there is seeing beyond looking.

So, what's the point? Why do this abstract, difficult and very esoteric practice of sustaining the vision of light more than form? It is the end of suffering and fear; the world becomes divine. In meditation with eyes closed we go beyond the darkness of the void to the light of the Self; similarly, in meditation with eyes open, we go beyond the changing forms to the light of the Self. We become established in the highest state—the contentment of pure being which underlies all other states. This is why we do this practice; to know our true Self.

We also do this practice because it is given to us by a master of meditation, one who is permanently established in the highest possible state attainable by a human in this incarnation. This teacher is perfect in wisdom, humility, purity and power. She gives us perfect love, guidance and inspiration. She will give us her state if we will only accept it. She gives us our Self.

We require a perfected master to teach us about our true self because we normally do not get this on our own. When we take form in this physical plane, our attention is distracted by sensory phenomena and we become entangled in the dream of forgetfulness. We must be awakened by one who is perfect in remembrance.

We remember that we have forgotten when we ask, *Who am I, and what is my true nature?* This sets us upon the path of turning within to reestablish the balance of vision.

But what went wrong? Where did we lose track? What was the problem? The wise among us say that the ego brings the sleep of forgetfulness, it is the ego from which we must awaken.

The ego has a noble origin but attains only delusion and must, in the end, be merged back into that which gave it birth. So let's take a moment and trace the lineage of the ego to put its emergence and fate into perspective. The ego has its roots in the underlying principle of all manifestation, pure Universal Consciousness. This primal Absolute Unity, also called

*Paramashiva*, possesses the potential for manifesting all that is ever likely to be, as well as the powers to differentiate and to know or survey Itself.

The immanent creative power of the transcendental *Paramashiva* is called *shakti*. The creativity of *shakti* causes the first differentiation of knower and known, of "*I*" and "*this.*" At this stage in the universal unfolding, pure consciousness is aware of itself. All potential manifestation also possesses this power of self-consciousness. In the following stage of development the veil of *maya* (illusion) is drawn as sentient beings on the physical plane manifest this power of self-reflection. Only, this self-awareness is limited to the local form while full consciousness of the eternal, all pervasive, and blissful Unity is concealed. This descent of differentiation gives birth to the ego: the psychic apparatus, that is comprised of intelligence, I-consciousness, and memory. The ego in this limited contraction of Universal Consciousness works fine for navigation in the physical realm, and for creating and absorbing *karma*, but the descent of differentiation must reverse course to become an ascent of merging.

The ego is redeemed by turning inward, becoming still, and once again attaining the state where pure Consciousness becomes aware of Itself. The knower knows itself, there is just "*I*" and "*this.*" The veil of illusion is lifted. The final state reappears when the experient and experience merges irrevocably into the eternal self-luminous bliss of Universal Consciousness. This is the Self given us through the grace of a living master.

It is one thing to understand that the ego is the cause of Self-alienation, but it is quite another to rid ourself of this pesky parasite. In our attempt, we find that the ego resists annihilation quite vigorously. So, let us put a microscope on the ego and reconnoiter what, exactly, is it about the ego that is so troublesome, and that keeps us blind, ignorant and self-destructive.

Previously the ego was described as the psychic instrument of intelligence, I-consciousness and memory. These principles of mental operation are also known as *buddhi, ahamkara* and *manas*, respectively. Our target here is *buddhi*, the instrument of ascertaining intellect. The *buddhi* sees the world as relational, that is, I — that. *Buddhi* is not the Seer, *buddhi* is the **instrument** of seeing. Universal Consciousness is the Seer. *Buddhi* makes a catastrophic misidentification. Patanjali tells us that, *Egoism is the identification of the power of the seer with that of the instrument of seeing.* [Yoga Sutras, Book II, Sutra 6] He explains that although the Self is pure consciousness, it appears to see through the mind. The Self **is** pure consciousness so when the Self sees the world, *buddhi* distorts the vision into a relational perception that there is an "*I*" in the body, separate from universal consciousness, that is seeing. This illusion of a separate "*I*" is the misidentification of the *buddhi* that is the ego. *To perceive the Self clearly, the mind must become very still.* [Gurumayi; Evening Program. Oakland 6/6/89] We see from this why it is critical to still the mind to approach awakening. When we become conscious of Consciousness in meditation it is self-evident that the Seer (*I*) is neither the mind (ego) nor the body. We grasp the Truth of the Kena Upanishad that says:

*At whose behest does the mind think? Who bids the body live? Who makes the tongue speak? Who is that effulgent Being that directs the eye to form and color and the ear to sound?*

The Self is the ear of the ear, mind of the mind, speech of the speech. He is also breath of the breath, and eye of the eye. Having given up the false identification of the Self with the senses and the mind, and knowing the Self to be Brahman, the wise, on departing this world, become immortal.

Now we know the secret. Now we know that the *I*, whom we always thought was this mind and body, is really the Divine

Presence. We can actually experience that it is the Divine Presence that behooves the mind to think, bids the body to live, makes the tongue to speak, and directs the eye to form and color, and the ear to sound. We awaken to the Self that sees.

The ego in its ignorance has imagined that it is a separate person from all the other persons out there. However, there is only one person. This Self enlivens myriad forms that exist as instruments of perception of the Divine Absolute. We may correct this error of mistaken identity by surrendering to the true Self, the source of love, light of wisdom, and eternity of bliss absolute.

*Let me tell you a simple fact. If you set aside your ego for a moment, you will realize that you, the traveler, are that which you are seeking. Everything is within you. The supreme inner stillness, the thought free state, is your destination. It is the Self, Consciousness. It is the Guru as well as the disciple. It is the Guru-disciple relationship.*

[Swami Muktananda; The Perfect Relationship, 1980. SYDA Foundation]

## The Goal

The one who loves us most wants only that we become free from identification with this particular person.

According to the Vijnanabhairava, the ultimate goal of yoga is identification with undifferentiated universal consciousness; also called the heart, nectar, Reality, essence, Self, or void that is full. This sacred text suggests four processes that are required for transformation.

1. Perfect absorption in the heart of the Supreme.
2. Passing from dichotomizing thought constructs to thought-free non-relational awareness.
3. Disappearance of the limited pseudo-I ego and the emergence of the Real Universal I which is divine.

4. Dissolution of the individual mind into universal consciousness.

This is the message as well as the state of saints and sages in all times and cultures; this is the one perennial philosophy and the one final state. The guru is the means, self-discipline and grace is the method, and the goal is already attained. Walk this way into perpetual happiness.

## Four Gatekeepers

*There are four gatekeepers at the entrance to the realm of freedom. They are self-control, self-inquiry, contentment, and good company. Self-control means keeping your senses in check even when they ache. Self-inquiry means whatever the thought, whatever the incident, whatever the matter, contemplate it. Contentment means that whether you receive a little or a lot, whether you receive everything or nothing, you remain content. And good company is you, no one else.*
[Gurumayi, Chicago 6/20/87]

We pass the gatekeeper of self-control when it is no longer an effort to keep the senses in check. When it becomes a natural preference to maintain the sweetness of the steady state rather than chase the senses into pleasure and pain, loss and gain, and shame and fame; we enter the realm of freedom. This preference doesn't come easily or quickly, but steady effort brings the steady state. Self-inquiry, contentment and good company all contribute substantially to self-control. Similarly, self-control gives much to self-inquiry, contentment and good company.

A further mastery that one must attain is contentment in the face of all that may befall us. It is to know *Ah, this is perfect* in every circumstance. Like self-control, contentment comes with a natural preference for the sublime serenity of our true inner nature over the distraction and disturbance of the everchanging outer drama. Contentment leads us to the realm of freedom as surely as our desires secure our bondage to the realm of *karma* and rebirth. Whether you receive everything or nothing, you remain content.

Gurumayi cuts right to the heart when she says that "[...] good company is you, no one else." The term *satsang* is usually given to mean, *the company of the Truth*. When our predominant state is serene and joyful, the Truth expresses through us and we find contentment and fulfillment in just being. We are our own good company. If our predominant state is needy or distracted, the Truth is hidden and we are not good company for ourselves or anyone else. The realm of freedom waits patiently for us to remember and to merge into our true nature through the attainments of self-control, self-inquiry, contentment, and good company.

The fundamental discrimination along the path of *Satya* (Truth) is ferreting out that which never changes. The dawning of the immutable appears out of the ephemeral darkness at the auspicious time for each soul as it makes its way to the fullness of Self-realization.

We may be shocked into the awareness of the unchanging by the touch of a Siddha Master, or we may attain it over a period of time in meditation as we delve into the space between the words or become immersed in the Presence behind all cognition. However it comes to us, we find that it is absolutely the same each time we surrender to that deepest Self awareness. The Truth is always and ever the same.

We know the Truth when we experience that simple, pure, sweet tranquility of our innermost Self. The power of discrimination brings us back time and time again, face to face with our Self. We become truly great in this remembrance. We become divine when we never again forget.

*The Upanishads proclaim:*

> *As one draws the pith from a reed, so must the aspirant after Truth, with great perseverance, separate the Self from the body. Know the self to be pure and immortal — yea, pure and immortal.*

> *The Ancient One is unborn, imperishable, eternal. Though the body be destroyed, he is not killed. The Self forever dwells in the hearts of all. When one is free from desire, his mind and senses purified, he beholds the glory of the Self and is without sorrow. These are the highest truths taught in the scriptures.* [Kena Upanishad]

If we think we are the body then the world is predominantly sensory; a constant round of pleasure and pain. If we think we are the mind, our life is largely mental and emotional; a roller coaster of feelings. When we discover that we are the Self, and become established in that divine Presence, we merge into the unchanging serenity of joyous perspicacity. This is living in the Truth.

~

Modern physics tells us that this universe that we know and love so well all began long ago and far, far away. We are to believe that fourteen billion years ago a condensed primordial singularity suddenly became an expansion of energetic radiance. There is little speculation among physical cosmologists as to the nature of the universe previous to the expansion because the laws of physics do not apply to a state of density where time, space and boundary cannot be determined. Whatever the precursor, it ignited totally and instantaneously into light. This was an extraordinarily high-energy and unfathomably hot event that rushed outwardly headlong into the vastness of cold space.

As expansion increased, cooling began. At the age of 100 seconds the universe had cooled by a billion degrees precipitating nucleosynthesis. Primordial nucleosynthesis occurs when photon propagation waves lose energy rapidly in the expansion causing them to curl up and contract into discrete packets, or quanta, of energy. We can get a sense of this fundamental transmutation of energy into matter by looking at its reverse. You may recall seeing bubble tracks of meson decay where the decaying particle spirals inward in its transmutation from matter to energy over a period of a billionth of a second releasing hundreds of million electron volts of energy. Picture a photonic wave curling up, transforming the energy of light speed into mass as it is chilled by a billion degrees.

This high-energy accretion and cooling of the primordial radiance formed three basic varieties of quanta: protons, neutrons, and electrons. These discrete quanta possess spin, charge, momentum and mass. They also form a natural relationship with each other, the most basic of which is hydrogen (1 proton, 1 electron).

Hydrogen is the mother of all matter. Heavier elements are formed in high-energy events where protons and neutrons are fused into the nucleus of the hydrogen atom. This increase in nuclear charge and mass draws free electrons into the orbital shells of the new element.

The total mass of the universe is predominantly hydrogen. Hydrogen propagates the carrier wave of the fundamental resonance, or vibration, of the universe. Some call it a reverberation of the big bang. This radiant energy broadcasts in the microwave band at a wavelength of ten millimeters. This corresponds to a temperature of 2.75° K. The temperature of the primal event was $10^{10}$K or ten billion degrees Kelvin. [Wilkinson, D.T., "Anisotropy of the Cosmic Blackbody Radiation," Science, June 20,1986, pp. 1517-1521]

In 1964, Penzias and Wilson of Bell Labs listened for the first time to the hum of hydrogen, the Cosmic Blackbody Radiation

(CBR), through a highly sensitive microwave antenna. But Penzias and Wilson weren't the only ones listening. The human sensory apparatus is composed of structure and function, brain and mind respectively. The brain is mostly hydrogen and the mind is a field of consciousness. If you think about it, it's not surprising that the field of consciousness should be able to sense the resonance of the hydrogen in the brain as it hums along with itself all throughout the universe.We all know that the right hemisphere of the brain has special abilities related to synthesis, creativity and intuition. It is here in the right hemisphere that the universal resonance is perceived. We listen for it when the consciousness is focused inward and the thought processes have been stilled, as in meditation. This is the inner sound, or sound current.

Paramahansa Yogananda, writing on the inner sound says, *Listen to the cosmic sound of Aum, a great hum of countless atoms, in the sensitive right side of your head.*

Yogananda wrote this long before Penzias and Wilson *discovered* the great hum of countless atoms. Yogananda gives here a meditation practice that has been given to seekers after Truth for millennia. Absorption in the sound current leads one directly to the highest state. To attain this we ride the wave of the sound to its source: pure consciousness. The sound is the resonant foundation of the physical universe, and we can use it to discover deeper levels of awareness.

Once immersed in the sound we expand our awareness in a great leap outward to merge into the silent witness of all creation. In this way, the body melts into the universe.

Heavy elements are born from hydrogen. Hydrogen was created from protons, neutrons and electrons, and these particles emerged from light. In the same way, consciousness is the progenitor of light, and infinite joy is the state of pure consciousness. The body melts into the universe. The universe melts into the soundless voice. The sound melts into the all-shining light, and the light enters the bosom of infinite joy.

Enjoy now the full text of Yogananda's meditation on the inner sound:

"Listen to the cosmic sound of **Aum,** a great hum of countless atoms, in the sensitive right side of your head. This is the voice of the Self. Feel the sound spreading through the brain. Hear its continuous pounding roar.

"Now hear and feel it surging into the spine, bursting open the doors of the heart. Feel it resounding through every tissue, every feeling, every cord of your nerves. Every blood cell, every thought is dancing on the sea of roaring vibration.

"Observe the spreading volume of the cosmic sound. It sweeps through the body and mind into the earth and the surrounding atmosphere. You are moving with it, into the airless ether, and into millions of universes of matter.

"Meditate on the marching spread of the cosmic sound. It has passed through the physical universes to the subtle shining veins of rays that hold all matter in manifestation.

"The cosmic sound is commingling with millions of multicolored rays. The cosmic sound has entered the realm of cosmic rays. Listen to, behold, and feel the embrace of the cosmic sound and the eternal light. The cosmic sound now pierces through the heartfires of cosmic energy and they both melt within the ocean of cosmic consciousness and cosmic joy. The body melts into the universe. The universe melts into the soundless voice. The sound melts into the all-shining light. And the light enters the bosom of infinite joy."

[Yogananda, Metaphysical Meditations, 1964, pp.35-36.]

As you can see, the way the metaphysical cosmologist looks at the universe is somewhat different than how a physical cosmologist might see it. Still, what they see, in and of itself, is the same. The mystic knows the universe directly; the physicist comprehends by deduction. The great hum of countless atoms is a fine example of this. Another example might be the origin of the universe. Metaphysics, however, begins before the emanation into manifestation. Physics cannot deduce a state that is without form and beyond attribute; cannot measure the unbounded timeless state of no place. Ah, but metaphysics fearlessly describes in rich detail the abstract cosmology of eternity before time, forces before energy, and existence before manifestation.

The mystic knows the fundamental fabric of the universe to be pure unbounded, eternal, self-luminous consciousness *(prakasha)*. A rational empiricist has no idea what the universal matrix might be, but as long as the money holds out they will build bigger super-colliders to break up neutrons into smaller pieces until the fundamental particle is finally discovered. Does this make you chuckle?

When confronted with *consciousness* as an issue, scientists refer to it as *the ghost in the machine*. They might agree that by some mysterious process, some organisms *develop* consciousness. Empirically we know that consciousness exists. If it exists, it was either created from something else, or it has always existed. The knowers of Truth say that consciousness has always existed, and that from consciousness this world was created. Light exists as a contraction of consciousness; atoms, a contraction of light; substance, a contraction of atoms. Great sages, who we know to be right about everything else, tell us that at the beginning of the cycle all manifestation existed as potential in the *Maha Pralaya,* the great sleep of dormant consciousness. In this state the Supreme and its power of manifestation existed in undivided unity.

Because it is the nature of the universe to manifest, the creative power stirred, awakening the transcendent and immanent aspects of universal consciousness. This first differentiation of subject and object, *I* and *this,* set in motion further differentiation of the knower and the known. As this process of differentiation progressed, the known lost its awareness of unity with the knower. Differentiation continued through the process of gross elements of materiality emerging from the unmanifest.

The Vedic literature of the east tells us that everything manifest contains attributes, or genetic constituents, of three qualities in various proportions: light, energy and mass (the gunas of *sattva, rajas,* and *tamas).* In the unmanifest the qualities are in perfect balance. The elements of materiality display a predominance of one quality over the others. For example, photons express primarily light, and protons express primarily energy and mass. Objective manifestation, we are told, is a polarization of the creative power of the Absolute and expresses in the evolution of the universe as a natural matter of course. This polarization of creative power of consciousness brings us to the point at which the physicist begins to be able to describe the universe.

The cycle perpetuates until the manifest begins to withdraw itself back into the unmanifest to enter again the *Maha Pralaya.* This sounds just vaguely familiar. There is good evidence now that dark energy will eventually stretch the material universe into dissolution.

The source of being is only unknowable to one who is not conscious of consciousness. To attain perfect knowledge of the highest wisdom, one merely retraces the path of the manifest back into the unmanifest; follows the immanent into the transcendent. Specifically, this means to merge one's separate identity back into the non-relational unity of the Absolute. The known is ephemeral and dissolves; all that remains is the knower. *I* and *this* ascend into pure awareness of being.

# Destiny & Purpose; Everything & Nothing

*Can there be NOTHING?*

For there to be nothing, there must be a conscious perceiver of nothing. If there is nothing for the observer to perceive there is nothing but the perceiver; and that is something.

If there were no consciousness, there could be neither something nor nothing. But there is consciousness, so nothing cannot exist. There will always be something: consciousness of something or nothing.

The Universal Absolute (Brahman, Prakasha, the Self, many other names) being consciousness, is omniscient, omnipresent and omnipotent.... Omniscient, because consciousness (immaterial intelligence) is the knower of everything; omnipresent, because there is nowhere that consciousness is not; and omnipotent because consciousness has the power to know itself. This is the fundamental miracle of existence—that we are aware of being aware. Amazing.

It is the Self that sees through your eyes, and it is the Self that looks back at you through the eyes of another. See the Self in everyone, look deeply into their eyes, and feel The Presence.

*In the Beginning... Vibration*

According to Vedanta Philosophy, between epochs of time, primordial to everything, is *Maha Pralaya*, the great timeless sleep of absolute unity. It is unformed, homogeneous, boundaryless, conscious being, that is in no place but is eternal and immutable.

This unity remains complete and unchanging, until... movement. Out of the unchanging, how does movement arise? This is mysterious. The sages say that this vibration (*spanda*) is self movement. Presumably this means that when it is time for the absolute unity to awaken into plurality, *spanda* appears. *Spanda* is generally understood as vibration, pulse, or quiver. *Spanda* arises because that is the nature of the primordial conscious substratum that phases between epochs of form and formlessness.

Let's look at just exactly what a vibration is. A vibration starts with an increase in potential; a compression. This compression also creates a compensatory rarefaction of decreased potential. The compression phase causes matter to aggregate, and the rarefaction creates separation of aggregates. The aggregates clump into greater masses, and the rarifaction becomes thinner. Vibration becomes a wave; with amplitude, frequency, and power.

But wait, how is it that matter appears? How does matter materialize? For this we must reach into quantum mechanics and examine the essence of empty space. Looking closely we see that empty space is a bubbling foam of virtual particles (or quanta) emerging, annihilating, and a few becoming real. At extremely small distances of the Planck Length ($1.6 \times 10^{-35}$ meters) there arises something out of nothing. Thus we can consider empty space as a quantum field.

What is a virtual quanta and how does this quanta become a real particle? Virtual quanta exist for a very short time and are not directly detectable, but their existence can be known from the effect of fields of the basic force interactions. A virtual quantum becomes real when it exists long enough to be detected.

It is useful to know that virtual particles generally arise in pairs consisting of a particle and an anti-particle. In a symmetrical universe, a particle and it's anti-particle will always annihilate each other. But oddly enough, in this universe, symmetry is broken; that is, over time, more particles are created than anti-particles giving us a material universe rather than an antimatter universe, or no universe at all. Why this is, and how it works, is a mystery.

Just what is the nature of these virtual particles; are they hadrons or leptons, do they have spin, mass, polarity? Empty space is known to have a native energy called *vacuum energy* that is the cause of *vacuum fluctuations* in the quantum foam of empty space. It is precisely these vacuum fluctuations that arise as virtual quanta. These are little knots of energy that spontaneously contract to form quanta. It is easy to see how these virtual particles arise then dissolve on impact with their anti-particles. As noted earlier, if a particle misses its anti-particle, it goes on to become a real particle amongst all the other particles in creation, joining in the vibratory dance of compression and rarifaction.

Everything that exists was either created from something else or has always existed. All the matter in the universe begins with these fundamental building blocks arising out of the quantum foam of empty space, building up to the ever-changing complexity we see in the world.

There are two kinds of stuff in the universe: matter and consciousness. We know that consciousness exists, so it is real; however it was not created, and is primordial to everything.

Consciousness is the knower of objects, but is not itself an object, consciousness is the subject.

Even *Pralaya* is a non-existent state of matter where the *gunas* (qualities) are in balance for the cyclic sleep between epochs of manifestation. Consciousness is the eternal observer, even of the *maha-pralaya*.

## The SimpleTruth About Enlightenment

We are already enlightened; but it is the veil of the mind that obscures the vision of heaven from the experient. We get glimpses of the enlightened state in meditation when we pause at the stillpoint between the inbreath and outbreath. We glimpse the Truth of pure consciousness in the space between the words as we repeat our *mantra*. We feel the upwelling of perfect joy in the utter stillness after *kirtan* or chanting the Name. So it is that our practices take us closer to liberation.

To "become enlightened" is simply becoming established in that state of joyous tranquillity where stillness of mind is the default mental state. The tyranny of the mind has been broken and the inspiration of divine wisdom guides one in every moment. It's not that the mind doesn't think any more; the mind is used to manage the logical and logistical functions of living in the world. The mind and its monkey chatter, doubt and fear no longer drives our actions or jerks our emotions. The mind is the willing servant of love, compassion, service and devotion to the immutable, eternal Absolute; our own inner Self.

## India

A few years ago I flung myself to the other side of the world to search all India for the highest possible holiness— and I found him. Sri Sri Gurudev Omkarnath told me many things, one of which was *The book is already written; our job is to turn the pages.* Our destiny awaits us in every moment. Our circumstances could not be any different — the pleasure, the pain, the place, the time. All perfect to most efficiently redeem our *karma*. We are witness to line, chapter and closing cover of this light drama. In the beginning we don't know that it will end, and in the end we will not remember ever having been.

So, what good is it to have free will, freedom of choice? *Iccha Shakti,* the divine power of will, is the instrument we use to forge a joyous and contented presence amidst the kinetics of *karma.* This state emerges gradually out of the commitment, self-effort and loving surrender along the path to liberation. Muktananda tells us, *Effort is more important than destiny for Self-realization.*

The only thing we can possibly hope to gain in this incarnation is release from the bondage to our desires that bring us back to this karmic snake pit, lifetime after lifetime. The only thing we take with us is our *samskaras* and unredeemed *karma.*

54

Final freedom from the wheel requires that the *samskaras* be exposed and the roots of impulse cut out. These tendencies are illumined through meditation. Once we are able to sustain the inner stillness, then we become aware of what disturbs the tranquility. We see our tendencies standing naked before the compassionate eye of the Self. Once revealed, the *samskaras* lose their power, dissolve, then evaporate. This process requires great discrimination, unrelenting vigilance, right use of will, and vision of the goal.

*Karma,* likewise, must be dispensed with, so that there is nothing left to attract another body on the gross plane. The quick and easy way out of the *karmic* shroud is to be awakened by a Siddha Master and follow the path of perfection to liberation while still in the body. If it is not one's destiny to merge with the master in this lifetime, *karma* can, at least, be arrested through right understanding, meditation, and following the observances and restraints bringing purity and nobility to life.

### We Create Our Destiny

Thus as we turn the pages of destiny we hold the key to the final attainment. For it is we and no other who write these pages with the pen of our own action and reaction. When we are no longer the doer then nothing further is written. Doership is surrendered when the notion of separation is abandoned and we merge into the vastness of all being.

Destiny, then, is what we create for ourselves through *karma,* and free will is our choice of inner composure as we go through it. But what about purpose; what are we doing here? Why are we going through all this? What is our purpose in life?

We may have goals in life according to our desires, we may strive for fulfillment according to our needs, we may seek attainment according to our talents. None of this, however, accomplishes our purpose. All the effort and seeking in the service of the ego is only to fill up an imaginary emptiness.

Loneliness, defeat, betrayal and debility may empower us to overcome deficiency and spur us on in pursuit of success and happiness. But is this our purpose: to get comfortable?

Our secret hurt is not our fundamental limitation. We must look much deeper for the source of our discontent, the relief of which illumines our purpose. First, the limitation: When we incarnate into the realm of time, space and form, we make the transition from the Universal Self to the empirical self. It is very natural to identify with this body and experience a sense of individuation from other forms. In this process we forget our eternal, blissful, and unlimited Self. This limitation is our fundamental ignorance. Our purpose, now, is to overcome this ignorance and rediscover the divine presence within, which has been there all the time. We see here that our life's purpose is to awaken to the Self and become established in that transcendent state of steady wisdom. This brings the end of suffering. Why couldn't we just come into this world fully conscious, wouldn't that be easier than having to endure the darkness of ignorance and suffering? From the point of view of a single lifetime it's pretty much a drag to go through so much trial and error before getting to *Ah ha!* Let's take this from the perspective of thousands, even millions of lifetimes as the *Jiva* evolves to its final reunion. The sleep of imagined separation is a perfect vehicle for the karmic dance to play out. *Maha Maya,* the creative principle, is the power of the Absolute to veil its true nature from full self-awareness. Chief ally in this collusion is *Matrika Shakti,* the constructs of the mind. The Self, the witness, hides behind the veil of imagination until — Boom! — grace descends. Grace, in its deepest meaning, is the power of the divine to reveal the bliss of pure consciousness within the experient. This is brought about either by natural spiritual evolution, or through the agency of an enlightened one whose service it is to bestow that great awakening.

Many incarnations of great merit may bring us to the touch of the master. If we are astute, diligent and devoted, we can parlay this boon of grace into a quickening *of karma*. It is said that the fire of meditation burns away lifetimes of accumulated *karmas*. The same is true of the *samskaric* impressions. The seeds of *karmas* and *samskaras* live in the subtle body and germinate in the mind. The mind (ego), with its desires and imaginary identity, feeds and nurtures these seeds that results in a bounteous harvest of cravings, actions and expectations.

Meditation short-circuits this loop of head-banging by cooking the seeds in the fire of *Kundalini Shakti* until they no longer can be germinated. It happens in this way: The deepest *samadhi* is a purely selfless state. This inner ambiance of selflessness is completely devoid of selfish, egotistical cravings. The empirical self no longer feels needy of appropriation to fill up its emptiness. The individual lives in the world fulfilled by the ever-flowing fountain of inner love, spontaneous joy, and serene contentment. In this way, no mind is paid to the residual impressions that will wither, die, and never again bear fruit. Purpose has been attained, destiny has played out and free will has remembered the bliss of being.

A popular writer on yoga philosophy said: *Let us not forget, this is a yoga of happiness.* As one who delves frequently into the yoga of seriousness, this remark caught me a little by surprise. But as I contemplated it, I saw how true it is. Not only that, but the immense practicality of this perspective changed the way I regard yoga and life itself. **Boom!**

Let us consider for a moment what brings unhappiness; and also, let's examine the teachings of yoga that transmute our concern to unbounded joy. Life in the nuclear age has focused our collective consciousness on the popular acronym "FUD"; or fear, uncertainty and doubt. Media fascination with the morbid and bizarre, as well as live satellite coverage of international atrocity, feeds us a steady diet of horror and death. Fear is our constant meditation and governs much of our life. Really; think about it. Hold this thought for a few days and look at why we make the choices and decisions that we do. Look deeply and see if fear doesn't play some role in how we manage relationships, select purchases, do our work, drive the car, lock the doors, plan our future. As we catch the eye of this insidious culprit who stands blocking the light of happiness, ask what is the true source of this fearful intrusion into our awareness. Isn't it the mind — regurgitating the images and feelings from memory? Isn't it the imagination — concocting a drama of what might happen?

The mind learns fear through constant repetition of threat. Yoga psychology seeks to inoculate the individual with beneficence. If the injection is successful, then the mind attains immunity to fearfulness because fear has been replaced by loving compassion. How does this happen?

Stilling the mind awakens a new awareness of joyous tranquility just behind the mind. If this state is within me, it is also within you. If I relate to you as the embodiment of that divine sweetness that I have discovered within myself, then I am less likely to be intimidated or angered by you. The vaccine has worked. We are both happier now that I see things a little differently. The inner Self is stronger; fear has weakened.

*Once the fountain of love is unlocked in our hearts, we see the magnificence of our existence. With that love we turn this world into a paradise.      - Gurumayi*

Even as you and I are expressions of the love of the Self; this world, too, emerges from the bliss of the Absolute. We are only afraid of the world that we imagine to be different from ourselves. Yoga philosophy teaches that when we see the world as the Self, then we are free. We have come to the end of fearfulness. *Et voila* The yoga of happiness triumphs over fear.

We are dealing with two levels of yoga here; one, the belief system; and two, the experience of well-being amidst the uncertainty and doubt of living in the world. Simply accepting the tenets of yoga philosophy eases the mind to contentment. For the most part the ancient teachings are verifiable in experience; therefore empirical proof of their truth is at hand.

Some of the fundamental assumptions deal with extremely subtle matters, vast concepts, or experiences beyond what we might confirm while still in the body. Even though these things may not seem immediately verifiable, they are logically consistent with the whole of the system. There comes a point where it is futile to struggle with the mysterious, as it serves us better simply to trust those great saints and sages who are right about everything else, to be right about the inexplicable. In this way, we gradually merge into the happiness that we seek.

Whatever it is that we pursue in the world, be it pleasure, wealth, power, status, or comfort, our truest innermost desire is for these attainments to bring us happiness. Right? Our strivings may or may not be successful. And if we get what we want that makes us happy, how long does it last? This is not something we didn't already know.

## Yogic Powers?

The happiness that springs spontaneously into being when the mind is content has always been there and can never be taken away. Isn't this the most practical means to attain eternal happiness? It's so simple.

Simple; perhaps. Easy; not very. One must have great determination and endurance to become steeped in the perception that the world is not different from the fabric of our own inner Self; so that we love the world just as we love our own native being, the guru within. Just as all *that* is me, I am all *that*— everything everywhere in all time. I am omnipresent. You are omnipresent, merged in all being; boundaryless.

Omnipresence sort of hangs out with omniscience and omnipotence. Maybe we can expand into being everywhere, but what about being all knowing and all-powerful? Can we feel the great authority of all knowledge and power? Sounds a bit inflated, doesn't it?

Consider then, that omniscience doesn't necessarily mean that we can recite the taxonomy of paleopiscetology or encompass the collected works of all scholars. Omniscience means being so clear that inspiration shines the light of Truth at every moment, and we somehow just know the right action (*Dharma*) that is perfect in each circumstance. When the mind is undistracted by its own contraction, then we are totally open to the wisdom of divine omniscience. Our inner knowing is far beyond, and much greater than, the deductive processes and emotional knee jerks of the mind. The key is the clarity of the thought free state. Once again — the contented mind.

To grasp our omnipotence let us first examine the five powers traditionally attributed to the Great Self:

1. The power to create
2. The power to sustain
3. The power to destroy
4. The power to veil Itself
5. The power to reveal Itself to Itself

Implied in the power to create is the creation of the universe. The universe is comprised of all that we perceive, and the creator is our own awareness. We create with our awareness not only the solid world of our physical environment, but we create (and recreate moment by moment) myriad universes in our imagination. Given that the world is an outpicturing of our inner creations we see the awesome power that we possess to create.We have the power to sustain all that we create through the focus of our awareness. In fact, whatever our primary focus, at the time of leaving the body, is what will be sustained into the next incarnation. Choose very, very carefully what absorbs your interest.

Just as we have the power to create the perceptible universe, we have the power to withdraw the universe and its constituent parts. The presiding deity of this power is *Shiva* who is known as the destroyer of ignorance. The highest use of this power is to slay the mind with the sword of discrimination. Discrimination in this framework means to differentiate the real from the illusory, the eternal from the ephemeral. The result of this winnowing is that only pure consciousness remains after the chaff of the contents of the mind is blown away. We have this power. We *are* this power.

The power of the Absolute to veil its perfection allows us to develop forgetfulness by becoming fascinated with the contents of the mind. The power to reveal this perfection manifests ias the discovery of unconditional happiness emerging from within. We exercise these powers through our will to focus awareness on the inner state of steady wisdom, or to focus upon the ever-changing dream of forgetfulness.This suite of powers constitutes our omnipotence. Taken together with omniscience and omnipresence we have no choice but to accept our own full and eternal divinity. Whatever obstacle that might arise in life can be transcended through the wisdom of inspiration, the power of discrimination, and enfolding it into a greater presence. To come into full ownership of our rightful heritage we must remember to practice seeing the world as the Self, listening to the inner inspiration, and using the full power of will to sustain the highest state. Yoga teaches that the Self dwells within you as you. This becomes fully realized in the unfolding of our innate omniscience, omnipotence, and omnipresence. Dharana 85 verse 109 of the <u>Vijnanabhairava</u> states: *The highest Self is Omnipotent, Omniscient, and Omnipresent.* Since I have the attributes of Shiva, I am the same as the highest Self. With this firm conviction one becomes Shiva.

*Inner Shiva*

Becoming Shiva implies perfection. This means that to take this yoga all the way, we shall become perfect. Admittedly this is a little different from what we are usually told about ourselves. For instance, did our parents tell us that we were always perfect just the way we were? Did my father say to me when I was five years old, *Precious first born son, your playful creativity of pouring a shoe full of sand into the gas tank of the man who has come to paint our house fills my heart with gladness.* Perfection was strangely absent from his vocabulary that day. And at the age of ten I pondered deeply the minister's pronouncement that we had been born in sin. This seemed somewhat an inauspicious beginning and left me a little discouraged. These little insults add up over time to leave an impression that perfection is just not for us mortals.

A friend asked, perhaps skeptically, *Are you going for perfection?* I threw her a red herring to avoid answering the question. In the moment I knew that either yes or no was not quite right. The answer is both yes *and* no. No, because that perfection is already attained. Perfection is the very nature of our true inner Self. It is imperfection that is unattainable. At the same time, yes, one must pursue perfection to purify the mind in order to perceive the perfection that has always existed and can never be taken away.

The great Chinese sage, Karma Lo Tsu, gives us this benediction: *May all beings realize the ecstatic transparency of their own minds.* Of course the mind is only ecstatic when it is transparent to the contented bliss of the infinite and eternal Self. This is when we are the same as the highest Being. This is perfection.

The perfect state is easier to talk about than it is to get to. Still, we have lots of little helpers along the way. All the divine powers are nice little helpers. Discipline in meditation is a good little helper too. Can't forget grace as a little helper, and love is a *great* little helper.

We have love everywhere in our life and we can use it to take us to perfection. Just think; we love our car when it is new, we love our sweetie, we even love our favorite outfit. When we turn this love toward the inner Self we find love looking back at us. It is as if Krishna is inside just waiting for the *raslila*, the play of love, to begin. From the scripture <u>Bhagavatam</u> the inner Krishna says to us:

*What ineffable joys does one find through love of Me, the blissful Self! Once that joy is realized, all earthly pleasures fade into nothingness.*

*To the one who finds delight in Me alone, who is self-controlled and even-minded, having no longing in his heart but for Me, the whole universe is full of bliss.*

*Those who only have pure love for Me find Me easily. I, the Self, am attainable by love and devotion. Devotion to Me purifies even the lowliest of the low. Without love for Me, virtues and learning are fruitless.*

*By thinking of sense objects one becomes attached to them. By meditating on Me, and dwelling on thoughts of Me, one experiences increasing love of Me and at last is merged in Me.*

*Let your mind not run after the things of the world, for they are as empty as dreams. Give your mind to Me, meditate on Me. Learn to love solitude and think of Me without ceasing.*

*The world of the senses has no absolute reality, for it perishes. Therefore give up desire for ephemeral enjoyments and live in the world completely unattached.*

*The Self alone is real. The world of the senses is super-imposed upon it. See the one reality, the divine Self, and so liberate yourself from thinking about the world of the senses. A wise person regards the body as only an instrument through the help of which, by meditating on the Truth and knowing the one existence, he may become free.*

*One who worships Me steadfastly with devotion soon attains purity of heart and finds Me dwelling within. When he realizes Me, the Self of all, the knots of the heart are loosened, all doubts cease, and he is free from the bondage of karma. For the yogi who loves Me and whose heart is one with Mine, there remains nothing to be attained.*

Love Krishna, love your Self; your life will be filled with love. Love of the Self is the path to perfection and liberation.

Swami Muktananda once said that *the perfect worship is to have nothing before you*. This gave me some cause to reflect. Usually we think of worshipping *something*... you know; money, God, the Dallas Cowboys: *something!* Worship implies reverence and devotion. It is not too great a stretch to revere a great being, or to be devoted to a spiritual ideal or path. But how does *nothing* fit in with worship?

We get a clue from verse 46 in the <u>Skanda Purana</u> that says, *the guru is without form and transcends all attributes.* We know that the guru is both the form and the formless, both the person and the state. In this case the form leads us to the formless. In fact, *most* forms intrinsic to spiritual practice lead us to the formless. This is true for the various deities, scripture, ritual, service, meditation, chanting, even the *mantra;* all are forms that lead us step by step to the goal of anchoring in that formless Unity, the life of all being.

A true guru has the power to awaken us to the eternal formless Truth within. Deities such as Brahman and Shiva represent that pure state of "just being" that we seek in meditation. Scriptures of the east commonly say that the nature of the Self is pure unbounded consciousness. Ritual worship or ceremony attunes us to the highest aspects of our inner Self. Service to the guru teaches us selflessness in the workplace. Meditation, it goes without saying, takes us to identity with the formless. Chanting the Sanskrit names of the nameless formless opens the heart to that formless state of love. The *mantra,* as subtle as it might be, still guides us inward to the most subtle and sublime sweetness of the Self. Swami Muktananda says about this:

*Syllables uttered aloud do not constitute a mantra. Indeed, mantra is the great Shakti who brings the syllables to life; it is the awareness of inner unity. The consciousness of unity pulsing within a seeker is mantra. One who constantly repeats a mantra with correct understanding is raised by its power to divinity. This is the purpose of mantra.*

Looking again at Baba's aphorism that *perfect worship is to have nothing before you;* this does not mean that *nothing* is empty. It is full of awareness, intelligence and the bliss of contentment. Nothing, here, means no - thing; no icon, no person, no past or future, non-relational, no imagination, no syllables in the mind, not different from the Witness: only the power, the knowing and the presence of formlessness. To worship *This* is the perfect worship. Reverence and devotion to this realm of the heart is the perfect worship, complete surrender to the vastness of bliss is the perfect worship.

All this ado about nothing is not unique to eastern culture. There have been great beings in the west also who have discovered that less is more until nothing is everything. Saint Francis comes to mind as one who, in the 12th century, guided his brother monks into divine austerity. To illustrate this profound simplicity he said: *That which you are looking for is that which is looking.* Could there be any greater economy of aspiration?

Perhaps more to the point of finding perfection in the fullness of the void is the wisdom given us by the 16th century Spanish mystic, Saint John of the Cross:

*To come to the knowledge of all,*
*desire the knowledge of nothing.*
*To come to possess all,*
*desire the possession of nothing.*
*To arrive at being all, desire to be nothing.*

Saint John is not just philosophizing here, he is pouring out the heart of his experience. He challenges us to enter his exalted state simply by attaining to nothing. For free, he gives us the key, paid for in unimaginable suffering, just so that we can have it all by letting it all go.

Any discussion of nothing and everything would be incomplete without the thoughts of the great contemporary avatar, Meher Baba.

*All activity everywhere in creation is but a play of everything and nothing. When there is a complete cessation of this activity the nothing prevails. When this nothing is attained you have everything. Relatively, therefore, the nothing is everything, whereas that which we call everything is nothing.*

[Meher Baba, The Everything and the Nothing. Beguine Library 1963]

Merging into the true everything can be attained by approaching it from two different directions simultaneously. We must, of course, practice reverence and devotion to the serene inner Presence that looks out onto the play of activity. We must also renounce our misunderstanding that we are this isolated, limited, helpless, and unloved person who is desperately attached to ephemeral things, people and opinions of the false everything. Essentially, we renounce the true nothing.

Renunciation, to some, means withdrawing from participation in the abundance of our world. Renunciates often take self-righteous pride in their severity. This approach to renunciation may not lead ultimately to liberation. True renunciation is surrendering limitation and attachment. In this way we live in the world in a divine state. As Gurumayi says: *In the state of the witness, there is detachment. People may be there, but you are not involved in their lives. Things may be there, but they no longer bind you. Ignorance may be there, but it is not a trap. You merge into the supreme Self because the Self is the witness.*

Becoming established in the witness state is cultivated in meditation and perfected while living in the world. At first we meditate on something. In time we can meditate on nothing;

but even this is focusing on something even though it is nothing. Eventually we must drop meditating on anything and just be *that which is looking.* Commentary on verse 106 of the Vijnanabhairava states that, *A yogi is always mindful of that witnessing awareness which alone is the subject of everything, which is always a subject and never an object.* This takes "us" out of the picture. We no longer see; divine Consciousness sees through us. This is the moment of merging, when we are no longer separate from the seer.

It is only the ego that imagines wanting something, or has expectations, or is dissatisfied. Only the ego loves or hates, grieves or rejoices, dies or takes birth. Our eternal being awakens from the long dream when the ego becomes the drop that dissolves into the ocean of unbounded Consciousness.

When the serene Absolute peers out of these eyes and sees Itself peering out of all other eyes, then we are immersed in *Chidvilasananda,* the bliss of the play of Consciousness. Even amidst the blathering of *vrittis* and dramatics of *samskaras,* we are sheltered in right understanding that we all are danced by the one Self who knows through all minds, sees through all eyes and loves through all hearts. When we see perfection everywhere, when we love the Self in everyone, we have fully sanctified our life. The work is finished. We are free.

# SELF Revelation

## Who Are You?

Some of my favorite imagery from the works of Lewis Carroll is that of the green caterpillar perched on a broad leaf regarding Alice as she makes her way through a place that is not Kansas anymore. Disregarding his hookah for a moment the caterpillar enquires of Alice, *Whooo are youuu?* in a drawl that just has to be taken seriously. Indeed, this question *must* be taken seriously; for the answer illumines for us the only Truth that we can know. Try it. Ask yourself. Now.

If you are reading this, then you already know that we are not the body, neither are we the mind. We are that sublime purity of divine presence that enlivens the body and lends intelligence, wisdom, and inspiration to the mind. But it is not enough to just know this. The knowledge is merely a superficial pacifier if we do not make the leap consciously to become the pure Self of all. How do we know if we have imbibed this perfection? Check the reality. How does it look out there?

The sages say that the outer world is a reflection of our inner state. So if life gets to be a bummer sometimes, let's take a closer look inside. Just exactly who is it that we really think we are? One who is attached to the stuff of the world will be needy and tormented by bondage. One who feels inadequate will be chased by fear and will pursue power. One who feels hurt will attract injury and will desire healing. One who is self-alienated will find rejection and need acceptance.

One who is Krishna will be loved by all. One who is Shiva is surrounded by reverence. One who is Lakshmi lives in abundance, and could Indra be anywhere but heaven?

So again; Whooo are youuu?

Once we experience the exalted clarity of the inner Self, it is easier to divorce the body from who we think we are. The mind, however, is a little more difficult because of the urgency of the emotions. Here we have to face the hard fact that, like the gross body, the emotions are of the lower nature. While in the grip of feelings our true nature is shrouded by the ego. We forget. Again.

We can use the turmoil to remind us to remember to return to the steady state, to expand into the love that wells up continuously from within. Then we look up and the world is perfect again; a perfect reflection of the perfect radiance of light and being; consciousness regarding itself with sublime joy.

### After Enlightenment... What?

Perhaps the simplest answer comes from Tibetan Buddhism; there is a saying,

"Before enlightenment I cut wood and carried water.
After enlightenment I cut wood and carried water."

Yes, this is true, but what is the meaning of enlightenment? Here it gets a little complicated, as 'enlightenment' is a relative term, and scales over a substantial range from awakening in the beginning to *kaivalya* at the end. We will start at the beginning. Vedanta philosophy says that to awaken we must still the mind in meditation; this brings the stillness of pure consciousness to the front of our awareness. We will call this, *knowing the Self.* It's easy to catch little glimpses of the Self as we sit quietly, but we do not approach full enlightenment until we become established in the inner stillness. This is a gradual process.

As we enter the path of yoga and meditation we notice a gradual inward turning. In this process we turn away from the disturbance of the world and begin to enjoy the sweetness and contentment of just being. This reflects a shift in identity from the ego, to the impartial witness of consciousness itself.

Looking out from the eyes of the Self, we come to live as the peaceful presence and follow *dharma*. Life in the world after enlightenment is the same as it always was, but our perspective has changed. We observe with the eye of the impartial witness. We no longer react from our conditioning; rather, we listen for direct knowing which shows us *dharma*, the right thing to do. We live as the peaceful presence. Fear, anger, resentment, desire, and ego no longer arise. We continue our work in the world, caring for our family, and practicing our *sadhana*. Or we could retreat to the forest; some do. It really doesn't matter; our state is the same in either circumstance. So, after enlightenment, life may be the same, but our way of seeing it has changed. We have become *jivanmukta*.

The Sanskrit term *jivanmukta*, is generally defined as *liberated while still in the body*. But what does this mean, exactly? *Jiva* refers to local consciousness that is not different than universal consciousness. *Mukta* means that the individual has attained *nirvikalpa samadhi*. The root *nir* means without, the root *kalpa* means thought or distinction; thus *nirvikalpa* means without thought. In *Samadhi*, identity is shifted to the Self, consciousness.

*Jivanmukta* is one who has become established in the inner stillness, is free from karma, has finished with the wheel of rebirth, and speaks from direct knowing. So how do we attain this state of liberation? In the beginning, we learn meditation to awaken inner peace. The essence of peacefulness arises when the mind becomes quiet; because it is the disturbance in the mind that causes our suffering. Through our practice we get glimpses of the stillness between the words, between the breaths, between the repetitions of the mantra. Over time this practice of inner stillness brings peacefulness in our life, and in the lives of all those we touch.

This still state arises as we separate the experience of pure consciousness from the stirring of the mind, as it is consciousness that is the watcher of the mind. When consciousness takes the form of the mind, it cannot know itself. As the mind is purified through meditation practice we shift our identity from the body, mind, and senses, to consciousness, the Self. The ego dissolves leaving only the impartial witness; watching.

The ego is somebody, the watcher is nobody. We make our way through years of *sadhana* to become nobody. The ego resists vigorously, but in the end the Self remains, and the emptiness becomes the fullness of *ananda*, the joy of just being. Absorbed in the Self through surrender, we can lose awareness of the body and mind, focusing our being in the most sublime state. This is the state that remains when the body falls away. We have finished; there is no return to the realm of suffering.

Like the *rishi* told me, *If you are in the meditative state when you leave the body, you may not notice.* This tells us that even our glimpses of stillness during meditation show us the eternity of our true being. Remember this every time you sit quietly. Feel it. Be it.

*From the Swetasvatara Upanishad*

The Vedas are the most ancient and most revered scriptural text in the world. It is a collection of revealed teachings by saints and sages from different times and places. The following quotation is from the Upanishads, the final teachings of the Vedas.

"The seers, absorbed in contemplation, saw within themselves the ultimate reality, the self-luminous being, the one Self, who dwells as the self-conscious power in all creatures. He is one without a second. Deep within all beings he dwells, hidden from sight. He presides over time, space, and all apparent causes.

"He who is realized by transcending the world of cause and effect, in deep contemplation, is expressly declared by the scriptures to be the Supreme Self. He is the substance, all else is the shadow. He is the imperishable. The knowers of the Self know him as the one reality behind all that seems. For this reason they are devoted to him. Absorbed in him, they attain freedom from the wheel of birth, death, and rebirth.

"To realize the Self, first control the outgoing senses and harness the mind. Then meditate upon the light in the heart of the fire — meditate, that is, upon pure consciousness as distinct from the ordinary consciousness of the intellect. Thus the Self, the Inner Reality, may be seen behind physical appearance.

"Control your mind so that the Ultimate Reality, the self-luminous Consciousness, maybe revealed. Strive earnestly for eternal bliss.

"The wise control their minds, and unite their hearts with the infinite, the omniscient, the all-pervading Self. Only discriminating souls practice spiritual disciplines. Great is the glory of the self-luminous being, the Inner Reality.

"Control the vital force. Set fire to the Self within by the practice of meditation. Be drunk with the wine of divine love. Thus you shall reach perfection.

"The Self, all pervading and omnipresent dwells in the heart of all beings. Full of grace, He ultimately gives liberation to all creatures by turning their faces toward himself.

"He is the innermost Self. He is the great Self. He it is that reveals the purity within the heart by means of which He, who is pure being, may be reached. He is the great Light, shining forever.

"This great Being, forever dwells in the hearts of all creatures as their innermost Self. He can be known directly by the purified heart through spiritual discrimination. Knowing Him, immortality is attained."

This is such a revealing passage, so clear and succinct. Best of all, I find it refreshingly consistent with my experience and feel an intuitive certainty of its truth. We are so fortunate, in that we are the first generation in history to have an English translation of these profound Sanskrit Vedanta texts.

## Karma & Dharma

The term *karma* is generally associated with the concept of reincarnation. In this, our deeds determine our experiences and whether we will finish in this lifetime (*jivanmukta*) or continue into the next life where we leave off from this one. Dharma is commonly defined as *attunement with righteousness*. Below we will discuss the relationship between *karma* and *dharma*.

Fundamentally, *karma* means that we reap what we sow. The way this relates to our life experiences is; if we intentionally harm someone, this action will return to us at some point in this or the next life (*papakarma*). Similarly, if we benefit someone intentionally, we will, in time, receive some benefit as a result (*punyakarma*). If we harm accidentally, or benefit someone anonymously, there is no karma in this.

So what does this mean for our life? Once we understand that everything that happens to us is karmic debt (*parabdha karma*) running out. The hard things in our life come to us as conditions we created with karmic actions. And the wonderful things in life show us our *punyakarma*. Obviously this is also true for others as well. When we see others in painful circumstances, it is their karma running out. It may, or may not, be dharmic to intervene with other's karma, as it may simply create more karma for us, and not really lighten their karma. We can not save or protect anyone else from the karma they created; just as no one else can hold back our self-made karma.

*Dharma*, as we already know, is doing the right thing. In the Vedic literature, there are numerous dharmas defined, but we want to focus on our self-dharma, called *svadharma*. Although, there is also family dharma, cultural dharma, work dharma, and of course *sannyasa dharma* for the monks. In our personal *svadharma* we examine the right focus and action of our life path, whether spiritual or secular. In every thought and action we can attune to our direct knowing of what is right. We don't have to rationalize with logic, or follow what others do; we just know. There is no mystery about this. We always know the right thing to do; the right path to follow. This is *attunement with righteousness... dharma.*

*Desires?*

Why are desires a problem? As we develop in our natural environment, desires arise as a natural process of living in the world. Desires are essential to live in the family, get an education, unfold a career, gain wealth and possessions. What's not to like about desires? They are fine for living in the world. However, we are so accustomed to entertaining desires in the mind that we just don't notice the real effect. We all know the essential teaching: *desire is the cause of suffering.* Is it, really? How does this happen?

First, let's just watch our mind for a few days. Observing the random thoughts that come up continuously like they always do; watch the desires that come up most frequently. There are four desires that make up a substantial fraction of our mind time:

Wanting something we don't have;
Having something we don't want;
Wanting someone to be different than they are; and
Wanting some thing or circumstance to be different than
it really is.

Suffering does not arise just because we think we want something; suffering arises because consciousness, the Self, has gotten hijacked by the constant chatter that is in the way of the serenity and bliss of the inner quiet. Having a desire creates an expectation that the desire will be fulfilled, and that will make us happy. The reality, in case you haven't noticed, is that desires generally end in disappointment, frustration, even anger. This dark state persists because of so many frustrated desires. What can we do? Gurumayi Chidvilasananda tells us, *When the mind sheds it's desires, it feels the peace and bliss of our true nature.*

We are already happy, content, and full of love; but where is this when we need it? Just behind the mind is the utter stillness of the watcher that thinks no thoughts, performs no actions. It is only the mind that is in the way of ever-present peaceful sweetness. If we can sit quietly every day and touch the stillness, that quiet enters us and eventually becomes our steady state. Wouldn't this be amazing, just to be happy all the time? Well, hard stuff happens in our lives, how can we be happy in the midst of pain or loss that is a natural part of life in the world?

Established in the steady state, we observe what happens, then we just do the right thing. This is following *dharma*. Life becomes simple and delightful; we look upon all life, even adversity, as perfect just as it is.

But what is this state? At some point in our practice of meditation, the mind will come to like the stillness. At first the stillness, being empty of words, seems to just be emptiness (*shunya*). However, once we become established in the stillness, we find the fullness of the emptiness. The sweetness that has occasionally arisen spontaneously, becomes our persistence experience. This is the nature of the Self, pure consciousness. We live in the world in the presence of this sweetness just behind the mind. At some point the gestalt will shift, the background stillness shifts to the foreground of our awareness, and the random chatter fades to the background. This is the final freedom. The mind has lost its urgency, and peace pervades.

I cannot resist a little trivia here on the Sanskrit word *shunya* that, in meditation circles, means emptiness. *Shunya* in the Sanskrit numerical system, is the number zero; and looks like this: "0". In the west, we get our alphabet and numbers from the ancient Romans, we all know this. But in the Roman Numeral system, there is no zero (a serious omission). In the 14th century (finally), the west reached into the thousand year old Sanskrit numerical system to fix this problem. Can you imagine a numerical system with no zero? *Shunya* has made a substantial contribution to the west, in many ways.

*Obedience*

It is not too great a stretch to get some strange imaginings off the term *obedience*. But obedience is a powerful aspect of *sadhana*. The perfect disciple is perfect in obedience. The perfect in obedience attains the highest. Swami Muktananda was perfect in obedience to Bhagwan Nityananda and Gurumayi was perfect in obedience to Baba. We each attain our own Siddhahood through this discipline of faith, surrender and power of will.

Faith, the inner conviction of the wisdom of the *Shakti*, propels us forward in carrying out the will of the master. Surrender is dropping the resistance to merge with the guru, letting the ego/mind dissolve to enter that state we share with the perfected ones. We use our power of will to overcome our limitations to follow the will of the master who takes us to unbounded awareness, eternal sweetness, and seamless serenity.

What is it that the guru asks that requires such conscientious obedience? The guru's basic job is to make us like herself, to take us to *nirvikalpa samadhi,* that is, to become established in the bliss of that steady, thought-free state. This is liberation from the mind and the myriad universes of its creation, including this world of pleasure and pain.

The story is told of the devotee who approached Gurumayi and inquired, *Gurumayi, you have given me so much, what service can I do for you to repay your great gift?* Gurumayi replied, *Meditate; attain the highest.* This should be a pretty strong clue in understanding what the teacher is looking for in the student. Obedience requires that we become steady in certain practices. Swami Muktananda tells us:

> *True Siddhahood means the state of being centered in the inner Self. It is for this reason that I keep asking you to meditate on your own Self, worship your own Self, honor your Self, do the mantra going on within you. Become your own Lord. Siddhahood is present within you in all*

*its power. You should only attain awareness of your inner perfection, your spiritual glory, your present Self. And you should stay in that awareness all the time.*
This is what the guru asks.

Faith in the virtue of these commands is probably easy. If we have touched the Self at all, then Baba's loving entreaty is self-evident. Surrender to the Siddhahood within is likely more difficult due to the persistence of naive information about our true nature. Most difficult, perhaps, is bending the will into the harness of obedience to maintain the awareness of inner perfection and spiritual glory all the time.

Fortunately there is not really any hard work to do about all this. All that is required is to repeat the *mantra* going on within, and all these other attainments just happen of themselves. We just let go and merge with the *mantra;* limitation falls away, glory emerges, and we float in the infinite perfection that was there all along.

In this way, we become initiated into a body of wisdom that leads us to the highest attainment. We learn that to obey the word of the master is the training we need to recognize the Truth, and the practice we need to immerse our forgetfulness in remembrance. This obedience at the feet of the master infuses us with mastery to sustain that state she has so lovingly graced us with.

Even though we resist, our conditioning will be burned away. Even though we rationalize, the mind will find repose. Even though we are disturbed, the heart will be swept away into eternal unbounded joy.

The Unchanging is the conscious being of all that is. The Unchanging is so unchanging that it neither comes into, nor goes out of existence. From the creative power of the Unchanging, emerges the mind that creates a diversion for the eye of the Self. This imaginary distraction is the illusion of that which changes. It is, in fact, a passing dream of the Unchanging and is, therefore, not real—a mirage of the ephemeral on the horizon of the Eternal.

We first experience the Unchanging not by its presence but by its absence. Its absence comes to us as the insecurity of being alone. We are like a rudderless boat being buffeted about, without anchor in the storm. The mind seeks everywhere for something to hold on to. Little does it know. We grasp at the ephemeral only to find sand slipping through our fingers. Happiness is a moving target.

Stop!

*In the kaleidoscope of change, seek only the unchanging.*

[Mikhail Naimy: The book of Mirdad]

The seeking instinct is inborn to all sentient creatures. We seek outwardly as a matter of reflex. However, the seeking must be turned inward to reveal the Unchanging. Of course, it is at the bottom of the pile of all the wonders there to discover as we turn inward. We can know the Unchanging, not by thinking about it, but by not thinking about it. We touch the Unchanging in the utter stillness of meditation. Here is the safe harbor where we anchor against the winds of change, tides of impressions, and storms of feelings.

We become the Unchanging through steadiness of character that reflects the inner stillness we practice in meditation. This is our home, our true nature, our source and goal. Here we find our Self; the end of our seeking and the beginning of perfect contentment.

The Universal Absolute, dimensionless and eternal, has within itself the power of creativity. Its nature is to alternate between epochs of quiescence and creative manifestation. To enter a phase of Self-expression, the Absolute creates within itself universes of dimension and duration that will again, at the end of the cycle, return to eternal Unity. This creation of space, time and form is a contraction of Universal Consciousness and is limited in power, knowledge and location. Sentiency in this limited universe possesses self-luminous conscious intelligence but because of its contractedness, does not know its creator.

This individual self-consciousness is, in fact, incomplete in its self-knowledge, power, and extent of awareness. As such, the experient feels a sense of incompleteness until the time of reawakening of the power of the Supra-causal to know itself. Haven't we all asked ourselves: *Is this all there is?* Don't we all want something or someone to fulfill us and give meaning to our lives? What is it that is really missing? What is it that will truly fulfill our longing?

What is lost is the full experience of unlimited consciousness and bliss absolute. But it is not really lost, it is only waiting to be awakened within. We might think of this transient ignorance as part of a cosmic game of hide-and-seek where the Self hides Its Self-knowledge in order to take form in this projection of time and space.

To illustrate, let's take the example of dreaming. When we dream, things appear solid and people appear real. What happens in the dream seems real, apparent pleasure and pain brings us joy or grief. When we awaken, we see that we have created an imaginary drama within our own consciousness and not any of it was truly real. In exactly the same way we shall awaken from the long-dream of this incarnation and realize that the vivid play upon the screen was merely a play of consciousness; whimsy of divine sport. The object of the game is to wake up before we die, or our fascination with the mirage will bring us back to the dream to pick up where we left off.

The question now is how do we shake off this burden of limitation to reveal the splendor of our true being. The sage Vasishta teaches Rama:

*When the mind is at peace and the heart leaps to the supreme truth, when all the disturbing thought-waves in the mind-stuff have subsided and there is unbroken flow of peace and the heart is filled with the bliss of the absolute,*

*when thus the truth has been seen in the heart, then this*
*very world becomes an abode of bliss.* [Venkateshananda,
The Yoga Vasistha. 11:33]

What Vasishta teaches Rama is what saints and sages of all
cultures teach seekers after truth and liberation: *attain unbroken*
*flow of peace.* Why this practice? What is so special about stilling
the thought-waves in the mind?

Mastery of this state mimics the consciousness of the soul
that has returned to its creator. When the body falls away
the mind dissipates. What emerges from the cocoon of form,
limitation and ignorance is full consciousness of the Universal
Absolute. As we mimic our ultimate transcendence ... *then this*
*very world becomes an abode of bliss.* Our soul becomes liberated
while still in the body, never to return to the dream world of
pleasure and pain.

Even though the heart has attained the Truth, nothing has
changed. As a Zen monk observed:

*Before enlightenment I cut wood and carried water. After*
*enlightenment, I cut wood and carried water.*

Life in the world goes on but our concerns over loss and gain
have melted into profound gratitude for living in the light of
boundless eternal joy.

### Great Beings

The foremost great being in the universe is our own inner
Self. Shiva, the primordial guru, is our own inner Self. Our
beloved Gurumayi is our own inner Self. Baba remarked once
that the **actual presence** of the guru dwells in the heart of the
devotee. So if our greatness is already attained, of what use or
necessity is a great being in our lives?

We have just one little problem: we are ignorant of our true
nature. We don't notice it at first because everyone else appears

to be enjoying the same ignorance; this is normal. The reason we are ignorant is explained in Sutra 9 of the Pratyabijnarhidayam. It suggests that the fundamental ignorance of our true greatness arises when the Universal Absolute, being omniscient, must become limited in order to take form. Thus limited, we do not experience our true perfection. Our inner great being is hidden.

An outer great being shows us our true Self. Think about it; isn't it common for us to have an inner experience of recognition when we meet a true Siddha master? We think the guru has something we want; but perhaps she has something we are.

One of the powers of the Self is *anugraha:* grace. It is through this power that the Self reveals Itself to Itself. A great being is the perfect servant of this power by revealing to us our divine nature. Grace is showered upon us simply in the being of a realized master. We can think of grace as *that natural force that causes the experience of merging*. Don't you find it utterly irresistible to merge into the tender sweetness of the guru? It is here in the rapture of surrender that we meet our own inner Self. For the guru is fully transparent to the Self within. She shows us our highest potential. How can we not surrender utterly to that true love that lives within us as us?

Strange as it may seem, sometimes it's easy to resist that natural force that causes the experience of merging. We stumble over our limitations, and often the mind leads us astray. The master is patient, always using the perfect means to take us beyond our ignorance and limitations. This compassionate relationship is illustrated in the story of the sage Vasishta as he gives instruction to his pupil, the avatar Rama. Now, the case of Rama is very interesting. Everyone knew that Rama was the incarnation of the Divine... except Rama himself. It was only after being instructed by the sage Vasishta that he learned his true identity.

We too are Rama. Steeped in ignorance, we only learn of our true nature after being instructed by the sage.

Surely it must have taken many lifetimes of merit and great longing to draw a great one into our lives. It seems such a miracle that we can sit at the feet of the master to imbibe the love, wisdom, and perfect serenity of a divine embodiment come to awaken us. How is this possible? What great calling brings an enlightened one into our midst?

These questions are answered by Sri Krishna in the Bhagavad Gita as he unveils this mystery to Arjuna:

The blessed Krisha said:

*My Self is changeless and unborn and I am Self of every being but using Nature, which is mine, by my own Power I come to being.*

*For whensoever Righteousness begins to fade away on earth, whenever grows Unrighteousness at once I send myself to birth. For the protection of the good, for Right to gain stability and for the wrong to be destroyed, age after age I come to be.*

*The man who knows my godly birth and understands my mode of deeds will never find another birth but after death to me proceeds. Relieved of passion, fear and hate, with me their refuge, full of me, many have come to share my state made pure by wisdom's austerity.*

*So it is that age after age, the eternal unlimited Absolute takes form to awaken Self-awareness in seekers after Truth. One of these forms was the 13th century Maharashtrian poet saint, Jnaneshwar. His exposition of the Bhagavad Gita in Jnaneshwari brought the light of Yoga to millions to whom it would not have otherwise been available. Following is Jnaneshwar's illumination of the verses quoted above:*

*By means of a mirror one object may seem to be two; but in point of fact, are there really two? So, verily, I am formless, O Kirti, but when I resort to the world of nature for a special purpose I behave as though I were incarnate. That I should watch over the strict performance of all duties and rites from age to age is but the natural course of the world from the beginning. When, therefore, unrighteousness overpowers righteousness, then I lay aside My birthlessness and, disregarding My formlessness, I become incarnate.*

*Then for the sake of my devotees, I take on form and, becoming incarnate, drive out the darkness of ignorance. Then I break the bonds of unrighteousness, tear up all the records of sin, and through righteous men raise the banner of happiness. I destroy the families of demons, increase the honor of saints and sages and unite morality with religion. Having removed the soot of indiscrimination, I light the lamp of discrimination, and then yogis enjoy a perpetual feast of light.*

*The universe becomes filled with the joy of the Self, righteousness dwells on the earth and my devotees feast on virtue. When I manifest Myself in the flesh, the mountain of sin is shattered and the day of righteousness dawns, 0 son of Pandu. For this purpose I am born from age to age. He who knows this is truly wise in this world.*

We see that it is the natural course of the world to manifest a great being in response to increasing fear, uncertainty and doubt. It is as if darkness beckons the light to manifest. It's a curious thing about darkness; no amount of darkness can banish the light of even a single candle. This occurs at a personal level as well as on a cosmic scale. If we become entangled in unrighteousness, it somehow just doesn't feel right. We seek relief from this discontent through purification, confession, or redemption through the grace of a great being. In this way, we seek out the virtues of our own inner greatness. When we see it reflected in the perfection, love, and wisdom of a living saint, we are inspired to release our suffering and its causes, and to follow the teachings and attain mastery ourselves.

Each of us comes to this point by a different path. Some, while leading a *normal* life, suddenly come face to face with the guru, and **BOOM!** Shaktipat. Others, after years of search and contemplation finally arrive at the feet of their destiny. No matter by which path we travel, we should know how to recognize a great being. Neither shock value nor erudition necessarily proves mastery. There are so many pretenders, how do we sort out the tangle? Is there a litmus test for the perfect teacher?

Shankara, the eighth century saint who brought the return of *dharma* to the east, tells us in <u>Viveka-Chudamani</u> the principal qualities to seek in a true teacher:

*A teacher is one who is deeply versed in the scriptures, pure, free from lust, a perfect knower of Brahman. He is upheld continually in Brahman, calm like the flame when its fuel is consumed, an ocean of the love that knows no ulterior motive, a friend to all good people who humbly entrust themselves to him.*

This is a very juicy passage; so let's look a little deeper at what Shankara has given us. **One who is deeply versed in the scriptures** means more than just encyclopedic recall. He or she is one who lives the truth of the scripture from the inside out. The *shakti* of a true teacher enlivens the scripture so that we receive the revealed wisdom of the sages into the subtle depths of our being.

**A true teacher is pure,** free from the impurities of *anava mala, mayiya mala,* and *karma mala. Anava mala* is the fundamental ignorance of one's true identity with consciousness and bliss. *Mayiya mala* creates illusory differentiation of Self and non-Self. *Karma mala* projects the misunderstanding of the separate individual performing good and bad actions. A pure one is in constant remembrance of the divine Unity and acts spontaneously upon the wisdom of the shakti.

*Free from lust* means just that. Additionally, we can understand lust as a symptom of the larger disease of craving in general. On this topic, Buddha teaches that, *If a man watches not for Nirvana, his cravings grow like a creeper and he jumps from death to death like a monkey in the forest from one tree without fruit to another.* [Dhammapada]

Craving arises innocently enough; we simply reach out to the world for something to fulfill our imagined emptiness. We just want to be happy. If we are lucky, we discover that pleasure is followed by pain, accumulation is followed by dispersal, and power is followed by collapse. The error of our ways is in expecting the world to bring us happiness. The wise seek inwardly for pure awareness of being, the light of inspiration, and the bliss of contentment. Thus the distractions of lust and other worldly cravings are sublimated. Happiness is attained within.

The teacher is a perfect knower of Brahman. He is upheld continually in Brahman; established irrevocably in the highest state.

The teacher is calm like the flame when its fuel is consumed.

Can you imagine what it must be like to have perfect inner stillness—all the time—*vrittis* nowhere to be seen? Isn't this what we seek? None but one immersed in serenity can give us this state. Such a being was Bhagawan Nityananda. About this inner stillness he said:

A person remains ordinary as long as he is led by the mind;

But freed from the mind he becomes a great saint. What is the use of many words?

Meditate.

You will get everything through meditation.

*... an ocean of love that knows no ulterior motive.* Hmm, you are saying to yourself, where have I seen this before? It was Swami Muktananda who taught us that: *Love is motiveless tenderness of the heart.* Motiveless; without expectation; tenderness; compassionate sweetness. <u>Shri Rudram</u> says:

"I will think only sweet and beneficial thoughts. I will do only sweet actions. I will select sweet things to offer in worship. I will always speak sweetly to both gods and human beings. May the gods protect me from any faults in what I say and make my speech graceful."

Not only is a great being motiveless and tender in love, but Shankara tells us that the teacher is an *ocean* of love; unlimited in vastness and unfathomable in depth.

Shankara asks that *the teacher be a friend to all good people who humbly entrust themselves to him.* This he should know about. Shankara had many thousands of devotees. His constant focus was to bring each one to liberation through spiritual practices, right understanding of the scriptures, and personal supervision of their *sadhana.* Shankara guided his mission the full length and breadth of India often with as many as three thousand devotees walking with him from place to place. He established several orders of monks that continue the practices and teachings of Advaita Yoga today.

Closer to home, Muktananda also has a prescription for the qualities of a great being.

"The only one who is truly awake is the one who has evolved from the state of limitation to the state of freedom. Waves of bliss of unity awareness ripple through that being. Such a one melts the ice of name and form in the ocean of Consciousness.

This is the awakening to knowledge received by the Guru's grace. This is the transcendental, the highest Shiva. This is the Guru."

Baba speaks eloquently and with authority on the state of a great being. In this passage he also reminds us that one who is free evolved from a state of limitation. We are all evolving, and many, through grace, have become free. We have looked at several prominent examples of beings who have attained the highest, but there are many, many more living life in the world who are quietly free. Their lifestyle may be unremarkable and their manner unpretentious yet they are truly awake with waves of bliss of Unity awareness rippling through their being. This is merely the natural outcome of following the ancient dharma of the Siddha path and opening to the grace of a Siddha guru. In this way our inner great being is liberated from the cocoon of limited perspective. It is inevitable that we will attain that which is already attained, in this lifetime or another. Perhaps it will help along the way to keep in mind what this is really about. Once someone asked Gurumayi, Why meditation? Why Shaktipat? Why a Guru? Why all these things? Gurumayi answered: All these things exist to shatter your dreams, so that you can enjoy the world as it really is.

# Final Transcendence

## Cosmologies, Relative and Absolute

The fundamental stuff of the universe, according to the mystics, is infinite, eternal, self-luminous, blissful consciousness and its inherent power of creativity. In its unmanifest state, this absolute being is dimensionless, in that consciousness and power do not constitute a dimension. It is only when this creative power generates movement in the boundless homogeneity that the dimensions of time and space simultaneously emerge. The objective relational universe thus comes into being.

Similarly, current scientific theory holds that our physical universe was created in a great flash of light out of the dimensionless unknowable, into time, space, and energy. These two perspectives have their similarities and their differences, and both are probably correct. Purists of each view are likely not very concerned with the respective alternative. But we regular pedestrians living life in the world, trying to manifest the divine presence out of an uncooperative mind, can integrate these cosmologies to experience perfection, here and now.

The mystic cosmology is the more comprehensive as it includes the physical; the physical cosmology does not include the ground state of consciousness in its scheme of reality. The problem is this: there is no reference by which the presence or absence of consciousness can be measured. Consciousness is indivisible, therefore cannot be sampled. It is non-relational, therefore cannot be compared. And consciousness is unchanging, so a gradient cannot be plotted. Yet, empirically we know that consciousness exists, that it enlivens all sentiency and that the pure experience of it across all individuals is the same.

Light is a common element to both views of the universe, however it is defined differently in each camp. For the physicist, light is an energetic wave or quanta of zero mass that is created out of interaction between charged nuclei or electrons. To understand the *light of consciousness* we shall consider the Sanskrit word *prakasha* that is translated as *light* in common usage and as *consciousness* in reference to the ultimate reality. Here, let us define *prakasha* as the principle of self-revelation or illumination by which everything is known. Consciousness is considered to be self-luminous in that it has the power to know or illumine itself. So you see that *light* in this framework does not refer to luminosity, as does physical light. In the Katha Upanishads we find that:

> *Consciousness is the supreme light. No physical light such as the sun, moon or stars or lightning shines there, to say nothing of fire. Consciousness is its own light. It shining, everything else shines in its wake. It is by its light alone that everything else appears.* [Katha Upanishad II ii, 15.]

Commentary on Sutra 1 of the Shiva Sutras says:
"Prakasha" is a most significant word that is not translatable into English, the word "prakasha" means "light," but it is not in the sense of physical light in which this word is used in Indian Philosophy. Prakasha is the light of consciousness by which even physical light is visible. Hence wherever there is any appearance, there is prakasha or presence of consciousness. Without prakasha (light of consciousness), nothing can appear, just as without physical light, nothing is visible. Every appearance is nothing but expression of consciousness.

[Shiva Sutras. Jaideva Singh, 1979, p 9] It was this *prakasha*, light of self-revelation, greater than a million suns that Arjuna saw after begging Krishna to reveal his true form. Saul of Tarsus also was transformed by this great light. Moses, too, was humbled by this light of divine presence.

Experiencing physical light is easy enough, but how do we know *prakasha?* It is one thing to be conscious, but quite another to be conscious of consciousness. We live not because of the body; this physical form is merely the earth vehicle for the spirit that moves it. Neither is *prakasha* the mind, although the unbidden tumble of imaginings is not different from the light of consciousness, only a contraction of the real. We delight in the full face of *prakasha* turning inward; mind bathed in stillness, our true nature is revealed—or at least glimpsed.

Even a glimpse is good. Remembering every day is better, but never forgetting is best. We do this because it brings contentment, happiness and certainty to life. It is the final fulfillment of life's purpose to live in the ultimate truth of being. We attain the highest purity to become liberated from ignorance, delusion, suffering and limitation.

## Paradigms of Truth

What could it possibly be like to become liberated while still in the body? How would it feel inside to just go about our daily business after having attained the highest state?

We have all met or at least heard about perfected masters living here on the planet, but typically they don't talk much about their own state. There are rare concise passages in the philosophical literature of yoga that gives some hint of the state and experience of a great being. The following excerpt from the Yoga Vasistha [V:53] gives us something to look forward to if we are persistent in meditation:

> *Purity, total fulfillment of all desires (hence, their absence), friendliness to all, truthfulness, wisdom, tranquility and blissfulness, sweetness of speech, supreme magnanimity, lustrousness, one-pointedness, realization of cosmic unity, fearlessness, absence of divided-consciousness, non perversity - these are my constant companions. Since at all times everything*

*everywhere happens in every manner, in me there is no desire or aversion towards anything, whether pleasant or unpleasant. Since all delusion has come to an end, since the mind has ceased to be and all evil thoughts have vanished, I rest peacefully in my own self.*

A great one allows us to see through his eyes for a moment to get a sense of the awakened state. If we look closely, we see that he also gives us instruction on how to follow the same path to perfection: we practice the virtues until they are our own constant companion, drop desire, attachment, and aversion; still the mind and rest peacefully in the inner Self.

First we have to figure out if this is what we want. If not, there are endless other diversions to occupy our time. If we do want unending joyous tranquility then we must follow the instructions. A sincere commitment, and doing the work, is the self-effort part of getting there. The grace of a living master is the assurance of finishing. Practically speaking, who could be a better guide than one who has already made the journey.

There is much more to it however than just guidance along the path. When one accepts discipleship to a Siddha master a link is forged, a subtle conduit is enlivened with spiritual power, a mutual devotion is entrusted for the liberation of the devotee. This shared grace not only frees one from the limitations of the mind and body, but the heart is opened to a wellspring of divine love. A vastness of true unconditional love is given us by the guru; we, in turn, return it to her and give it freely to all we touch. It feels so great to be immersed in love so fully and so completely. This is the love that endures through eternity. This is the nectar of our Self.

The mind enters the path to know the truth. The body enters the path to contribute stillness to meditation. The heart enters the path to lose itself in the rapture of its own love.

There are complete yogas for each of these three paths of spiritual advancement. Naturally there are also yogas that integrate the paths of the body, mind, and heart. The yogas of the body bring health and well being to the enlivened form. The discipline culminates in the practice of sustaining *asanas* in stillness for a period of time. The mind cannot cease its movement until the body is steady and comfortable in stillness. *Pranayama,* as a practice in *hatha* yoga, similarly culminates in the stillness of *prana* when one can sustain the attitude of the stillpoint between inhalation and exhalation.

*Jnana* yoga discriminates the real from the illusory and brings one to the awareness that all this is *Brahman,* the Self. When desire and attachment have been overcome and the mind rests in utter serenity, when the egosense dissolves into absolute consciousness, then one is liberated from the wheel of death and rebirth. It is truly an amazing thing to become fully conscious of one's own soul, then to reach further to become lost in the vastness of sublime bliss. Could there be anything more than this?

Yes.

There is another way.

Shankaracharya says, *Among all means of liberation, devotion is supreme.* [Viveka-Chudamani, "The Disciple" p.36- 37] Where the yogas of the body and mind are rigorous and arduous, all that the yoga of the heart requires is great longing for divine love. *Bhakti* yogas such as the Sufis and the Krishna cults take as their primary practices chanting the names of deities, worship of a god-head personality (Ishwara, Krishna or the guru), *puja, seva,* and *satsang.* The devotee becomes totally absorbed in longing, worship, service, and surrender to divine love. The following passage from Meher Baba lucidly illustrates the logic of *Bhakti* yoga:

> *God is Love. And Love must love. And to love there must be a Beloved. But since God is Existence infinite and eternal there is no one for Him to love but Himself. And*

*in order to love Himself He must imagine Himself as the Beloved whom He as the Lover imagines He loves.*

*Beloved and Lover implies separation. And separation creates longing; and longing causes search. And the wider and the more intense the search the greater the separation and the more terrible the longing.*

*When longing is most intense separation is complete, and the purpose of separation, which was that Love might experience itself as Lover and Beloved, is fulfilled; and union follows. And when union is attained, the Lover knows that he himself was all along the Beloved whom he loved and desired union with; and that all the impossible situations that he overcame were obstacles which he himself had placed in the path to himself.*

*To attain union is so impossible difficult because it is impossible to become what you already are! Union is nothing other than knowledge of oneself as the Only One.* [Meher Baba. The Everything and the Nothing." The Lover and the Beloved" p.1] Gurumayi, speaking on devotion, said that, *When there is love and nothing but love, what else can there be but total absorption in the Supreme Self.* [Evening Program 5/30/89]

Thus we see that there are several paths that can liberate the seeker from bondage to the world of suffering and rebirth, as well as bring contentment and the bliss of the Self to constant remembrance. There is, however, only one means to resolve the conundrum of pride and attainment. It is possible through self-effort, to overcome the limitations of envy, jealousy, anger, and lust; but pride is subtle as well as insidious. One may even become proud of attainments of devotion and surrender. Pride supports the egosense (which must go) and maintains the fundamental ignorance of our true identity. When I have attained something *I* am still separate from my Self. Only a finished master can make a finished master. Such a one, only, can annihilate pride and deliver the final attainment. The way we attain liberation is to take the hand of one who is already liberated.

~

A fundamental urge is at the root of all life: to seek nourishment. We see this from fungus to fragrant sandalwood, from paramecium to *this* peculiar species of vertebrates. This perpetual activity of outward seeking sustains life and drives social culture.

When the seeker seeks the source of seeking, pure consciousness emerges from behind the veil of imagination. The truth of the reality is finally made clear. We are no longer stupefied by the dramatic excesses of the ego; the mind no longer obsesses over its own contents. The personal identity of the observer falls away and the observed appearance simply is. We become liberated from the captivity of ignorance.

We see, on the physical plane, the magnificence of a Banyan tree, sleeping; neatly coiled in the potential of its tiny seed. When it is time to awaken, the seed spirals outward in every direction seeking earth, air, light, and water. At the end of its magnificence, it is dispersed back into the elements that made it — leaving only seeds.

At a subtle level, we too emerge from a seed: a seed *of karma*. When it is time to awaken, this germinal *karma* takes a body... a husk of earth, air, light and water. At the end of its magnificence, the husk disperses leaving only karmic seeds, thus perpetuating our suffering.

The seed within the seed waits, neatly coiled, for its time to awaken. *Kundalini shakti* opens the eye of Self-recognition. Seeing the perfection of divinity everywhere cooks the seeds of karma leaving only a burnt string.

This awakening of spirit resolves for us the mystery of existence and shows us our true Self. For this to happen, however, the impulse of seeking has to be turned within. Seeking within flies in the face of instinct that has insured survival from the deepest roots of our biological being. It is no small attainment to overcome the compelling urge to seek outwardly for everything and turn to face the great unknown. The moment comes when there is a shift in our direction. We turn away from the urgency to perpetuate another round of physical existence and turn toward transcendence of the gross plane altogether, to realize our blissful, eternal, self-luminous Self.

Only the mind is in the way of liberation. When we pierce the veil of the mind the unlimited dimension of pure awareness appears. Mental imaginings become more transparent to the groundstate of consciousness; we begin to feel the divine presence in our lives. To become established in the loving and compassionate state of pure freedom, we return again and again to the inner stillness.

*Om Shanti Shanti Shanti.* We see this frequently in the sacred literature of the east. We sing it chanting the names of nameless formless. Great beings offer it in benediction. Why? And what does it mean?

Shanti... peace. Shalom... peace.

Dona nobis pachem... peace.

*Om Shanti* is a universal injunction to turn our awareness toward the source of peace; and peacefulness is the key to heaven in any culture, in any age. There is a deeper purpose in all this to-do about peace than just wanting a friendlier world. Vasistha teaches Rama in the <u>Yoga Vasistha</u>: [II, 12].

*When the mind is at peace and the heart leaps to the supreme truth, when all the disturbing thought-waves in the mind-stuff have subsided and there is unbroken flow of peace and the heart is filled with the bliss of the absolute, when thus the truth has been seen in the heart, then this very world becomes an abode of bliss.*

Attaining unbroken flow of peace leads us to a realm beyond the mind and body, beyond even this universe of dimension and duration. We enter a state that was present before we entered this incarnation and will endure even when the body falls away. One writer on Yoga suggests that if we become established in that sublime tranquility, we may not even notice it when we die. All of Yoga is preparation for the last moment before — and the first moment after — leaving the body.

So, what's it like... leaving the body? From my own experience I will tell you that it is a rush into serene vastness. It's not as if a great expanse opens up and you are alone in the dark. You *become* the boundaryless serene vastness—all of it. You embody the infinite, eternal, self-luminous existence, consciousness, and bliss absolute. From this it seems only logical that if we reach out to embrace this state through meditation while still in the body that we merge with the Absolute for eternity. Similarly, if we never relinquish our identity with, and attachment to, the body and other ephemeral stuff, we will follow that attachment back into another body for yet another round on the karmic wheel.

*Om Shanti* is an invitation to merge more deeply into the serene vastness that is our true nature and is here at the end of the mind. It is also an invitation to release the fatal attraction to our mind and body, to say nothing of the minds and bodies of others.

Clutching this attachment is a sure way to attain death. Surrender to the peace that passeth understanding is a sure way to enter the boundaryless eternal Self. Pretty simple, isn't it? The path of Truth is the path of discrimination. Discrimination is the power to know true reality from the illusion conjured in the mind by our beliefs, expectations, and interests. These are the *samskaras* that constitute our ego. Our characteristic beliefs, expectations, and interests are created from attachment, aversion, compulsions, identification, addiction, and inhibition. These are the six deadly sins.

Great saints in all times have taught the importance of overcoming these six tendencies. But why? What purpose is served by releasing attachment and aversion; giving up addiction and compulsion; turning away from identification and inhibition? Is this just moral purification so that someday we may become proud of our attainment? Is this mental purification so that we might find happiness free from the conditioning of the mind? Is this spiritual purification so that our inner eye might look out on the world and see everything as it truly is? Is there something far deeper that is occurring as we discipline ourselves over a lifetime of practice to free ourselves of accumulated conditioning?

By transcending the *samskaras* of belief, expectation, and interest, we prepare ourselves to take the final breath and face the vast unknown. Typically we meet new situations with old conditioning. In the transcendent moment, we must be wide awake, fully open, totally present and adept at merging into Universal Consciousness. *All of yoga is preparation for the last moment before, and the first moment after, leaving the body.* Every time we sit for meditation is rehearsal for merging into the Self.

Liberation in this lifetime while still in the body simply means that we are fully prepared for the body to fall away; that we have already gone across. The Sufi Master Hazrat Inayat Khan once instructed his disciples: *Die before death.*

Once we know our true Self we see that we simply wear this body like a suit of clothes. Valmiki's Yoga Vasishtha [V:40] puts it this way; *Even though you are in a body, since you do not have the body, you are bodiless. You are the observer which is immaterial intelligence.* Surely your own experience verifies this to be the case. Valmiki states further that: *Death is but waking from a dream.* It is this dream that we must put away. The mental constructs of beliefs, expectations, and interests keep this dream alive and we will not awaken until the dream fades away.

~

Since childhood three questions have gnawed at me begging to be answered: 1) What is the nature of reality—the indisputable truth of being, 2) What are the means for experiencing the fullness of this indisputable truth, and 3) Who am I and what is my true nature?"

There are many who have opinions about the nature and cause of that which appears before us, but those opinions arise because of the disputatiousness of the mind. It is unlikely that we will arrive at indisputable truth with the mind projecting imaginary constructs into the discernment. To go beyond the mind and embrace the validity of our own pure awareness of all that is, is the hard part. After awakening to the ever-present Truth, the easy part is recognizing the self-evident wisdom given to us by the saints and sages, whose love is selfless and pure.

It is one thing to glimpse the vastness of serene bliss and quite another to become established in the immutable, eternal, unchanging Absolute. Therefore we require a means to attain this subtle state.

It is often said that: "The guru is the means." The guru gives us right understanding of what is really going on here. The guru gives us the practices that discipline us, immerse us, and free us. The guru gives us the grace to complete our return to the divine purity that is our true nature.

*Who am I and what is my true nature* is not a question that can be answered through erudition. The answer must be experienced in the utter stillness that reveals the indweller. This is the awakening for which we have taken this incarnation.

This utter stillness, given life by meditation, illumines the Self. When the mind is still, and the body is still, we have a conscious experience of the Self; of being the Self.

It becomes evidentially clear that we are not the body. The seer is the intelligence of the mind, and is not different from the Self. This individual, *Atman,* is possessed of *samskaras* bequeathed by the body senses and the mind (which is ephemeral like the body). As long as the ego is seriously interested in the drama of the mind and the pleasure or pain of the body, it will hunger for mental and sensory impressions after consciousness leaves the body. This hunger draws another body to go around again on the wheel of *karma*.

To purify the Atman of this blemish, we embrace spiritual disciplines to awaken and sustain the light of the Self. We love the guru to love the Divine in ourselves. We surrender to the bliss of the Self to turn away from the appetites that bring us pain lifetime after lifetime.

The Self is alive with power, joyous equanimity, and purest love. Our true Self is also wrapped in layers of imaginary identities. We must see who we are before we can know who we're not. But hey, once our eyes are opened to the eternal Truth, what's the point of continuing the charade that we are perishable flesh and imaginary ego.

Once the mind is purified of the illusion, the imaginary separation dissolves. We merge finally into our true Self. Through the grace of the master we do this while still in the body.

## Deities, Avatars, and the Conscious Substratum

Genetic research shows that about 40,000 years ago the primary diaspora from Africa to India occurred; and from there to the rest of Asia. From this we see that Indian culture is quite ancient. Not only is it ancient, the culture is contiguous over time with defining Vedic literature dating from about 3,500 years ago. This literature defines cultural structure and function including concepts of social *dharma* and transcendent philosophy, which continues to develop today. These concepts of *dharma* and consciousness are utterly unique to this cultural philosophy.

Let us compare and contrast Indian culture with western culture. Of course the defining diaspora to the Americas from

England and Europe could not be more different. The migration happened only 600 years ago, and cultural experimentation was brought here by many who had turned away from traditional English and European dogma. Yet much fundamental social and religious dogma survived the trip across the pond.

One aspect of Vedic culture and literature that is completely unknown in the west is the zoo of imaginary deities. Let's look at what this is all about. There are three classes of deities. Most are representations of particular qualities. For example; Ganesha the elephant god is known as the "Opener of the Way." For many Hindus, Ganesha is the family deity because he is the provider of everything. Saraswati is the goddess of wisdom and knowledge. Educational initiatives frequently revere Saraswati, including monastic orders. Hindus often pray to whatever deity has the quality one wishes to acquire.

Another class of deities can be thought of as avatars; these are the teachers of ancient wisdom. They are depicted in epics as the gurus of royalty and warriors. Rama and Krishna are the best known avatars who, in the literature, bring enlightenment to students like Lakshmana and Arjuna. Even though Rama and Krishna bring awakening to those lost in the darkness of ignorance, their styles are quite different.

Krishna manifests different attributes at each stage of his life. As a baby he is characterized as mischievous and unruly. As a young man he was the mysterious darling of the *gopis*. In his maturity he is portrayed as the guru and charioteer for Arjuna, patiently teaching him warrior dharma and how to know his divine nature. In other literature such as Srimad Bhagavatam of Veda Vyasa, Krishna is cast in a remarkable way. Krishna is given the voice of the Self. As Krishna teaches his student Uddhava, he speaks as the inner Self. It is as if our own consciousness is standing outside of ourself and showing us our innermost nature. We too are the disciple of Krishna; and what we read of his teaching is our own divine Self speaking to us.

Rama is unusual in that he was likely a real person. The story goes that he was born in Ayodha, became king and ruled with peace, prosperity and justice. He is the historic model of perfection in *dharma*. Rama was taught by the sage Vasistha, which is narrated by Valmiki in the six volume Yoga Vasistha. He gave these teachings to his brother Lakshmana, recorded in the original Ramayana of Vasistha.

In the third class of deities is Brahman, the nameless formless. Brahman is pure universal consciousness. There are no representations of Brahman, no stories, no drama, no teachings. Brahman is the conscious substratum of the universe, boundaryless, infinite, and eternal. While we are the local address of universal consciousness, Brahman is the universal address. We know Brahman when the mind is still; we know the ego when the mind is moving. It's one or the other. We choose. In this universalist class of deities we also have Vishnu and Shiva along with Brahman. Vishnu is the sustainer in the changing universe. Shiva is the destroyer of ignorance; thus is the deity of meditation.

All this development of culture, myth, and mysticism took thousands of years. How are we in the west ever going to understand the depth of the Indian culture? When we use the English language to translate Sanskrit, it is nearly impossible because English is a reflection of the western culture, and Sanskrit reflects a way of thinking that is not native to the west.

The way to avoid the language problem is to have a teacher with inner stillness; to practice the stillness of meditation; and to apply this stillness to our worldly *dharma*. In this, we simply live as the Self.

## Who Is The Guru?

The guru is one who attains to spiritual perfection with the power to transmit the highest state to another, and is given this power by another guru. This is the guru in form, but the true guru is formless. Beyond the form the guru is the grace bestowing power; this is the Guru Principle. Grace here means, *that natural force that causes the experience of merging.* This is the guru in principle, but who is the guru that we merge with in our final attainment as seekers on the path to liberation? What divine presence awaits us in our ultimate surrender? What is our experience when the guru is revealed as our true inner Self?

We are told that the guru and the Self are one; they are the same. What is the same is that each expresses as pure consciousness. So it is consciousness that is at the root of ultimate transcendence. The fundamental ground-state of being is non-relational consciousness, the Supreme Self surveying Itself, the subject void of object.

Here is the True Guru: more than a person, the guru is a state; more immediate than a principle the guru is an experience. The guru is our own awareness of being, bliss of pure consciousness, subject void of object.

## The Simple Truth About Enlightenment

We are already enlightened; but it is the veil of the mind that obscures the vision of heaven from the experient. We get glimpses of the enlightened state in meditation when we pause at the stillpoint between the inbreath and outbreath. We glimpse the Truth of pure consciousness in the space between the words as we repeat our *mantra.* We feel the upwelling of perfect joy in the utter stillness after *kirtan* or chanting the Name. So it is that our practices take us closer to liberation.

To "become enlightened" is simply becoming established in that state of joyous tranquility where stillness of mind is the default mental state. The tyranny of the mind has been broken and the inspiration of divine wisdom guides one in every moment. It's not that the mind doesn't think any more; the mind is used to manage the logical and logistical functions of living in the world. The mind and its monkey chatter—doubt and fear—no longer drives our actions or jerks our emotions. The mind is the willing servant of love, compassion, service, and devotion to the immutable, eternal Absolute; our own inner Self.

The Avatar Meher Baba teaches seekers: *Love God and become God.*

Typically in the west God is considered as some magical being separate from the believer and in some religions can only be reached through an intercessor. This puts God at some distance in this life and even in heaven. In this system, becoming God is unthinkable.

If God is truly attainable, what does the saint mean by *becoming God?* We begin this inquiry by understanding what is the nature of God. The Upanishads tell us quite simply: *What is God? God is the witness of the mind. God is that which knows what the mind is thinking.* We see here that God is not a personage or anything discrete at all. God is the ground-state of being shared by all sentient beings. All who see, observe. Consciousness is the seer, the observer. The mind, a contraction of pure consciousness, entertains itself spinning word pictures onto the screen of the mind's eye. This is so absorbing that an identity of doership emerges in the drama. This is where we get lost.

We get found by backing up to the step just before *spinning word pictures.* We can turn the inner eye of the witness to the utter serenity of just being, away from the futile chatter of the mind and the importance of the supposed doer. In this equipoise, the heart experiences the joy and wonder of self-luminous inspiration and merges into timeless unbounded transcendence. We become the nameless formless by remembering who we were before getting distracted by the senses. We become the Self by living the radiance of perfect peace, compassion, and virtue. We become the Self when separation dissolves, and there is only the watcher seeing out of all these pairs of eyes.

The difference between the guru and the disciple is that the guru is not troubled by the mind. Some wise acharya proclaimed, *The substance that makes up time is karma.* Everything that happens, happens in time. No time - nothing happens. *Karma* is fueled by unresolved attachments of previous incarnations. *Karma,* therefore, is the destiny of the soul. When *karma* burns up, time burns up. The soul is purified of its separate identity and merges into the seamless bliss of pure consciousness. So who is the doer of deeds?

Among the world's sacred texts there are a couple that are amazingly terse and profound: the Upanishads and Valmiki's Yoga Vasistha. Even though they are truly enlightened scriptures, they merely point the way. It is best to have the touch of a finished master to experience the state of divine realization. Thus the goal of the mystic is fully attained.

If we closely examine our experience of just being, we discover an awareness of knowing our surroundings illumined by the consciousness of the knower. Upon further investigation we find that this consciousness is present in the waking state, showing us our surroundings; the dream state, watching and remembering our dreams; and even in deep sleep, waking us to an unfamiliar sound.

This consciousness is our sentiency, our aliveness. It is the in-dweller, the observer. It is the Self of our self. The self-luminous indweller is its own light of consciousness and is intelligent: it knows what it sees. Furthermore, it knows itself.

This self-luminous intelligence is the Universal Verity, all else being merely contractions of this sea of primal bliss.

The witness through these eyes is just such a contraction, imagining separation. The disjunction is resolved when the eye of the witness turns within to its source. It sees the light of utter equipoise. This is the trail back home.

Odd that this self-evident truth is not self-evident until one who knows enlightens us. Then we say: *Oh, indeed, this is my experience. This is my true Self. How did I miss it before?* It can only be the mind's unending infatuation with its own contents that obscures the eternal and unchanging bliss of the

Self. Through purification of the mind, the seer transcends the obfuscation of the mind, and its own Self is revealed. This radical and profound shift in content liberates us from limitation and awakens us to our own divine nature. It is also through this discovery that we know the source of our sentiency — the Universal Absolute, or any name for the Divine we care to put to it.

*Permanence and Impermanence*

We experience the changing all the time. We can also experience the unchanging under special conditions. Notice the experience when the mind is still in deepest and most serene meditation. Notice also that each time this state is returned to, it is the same; it does not change. Over time this state is found to be the unchanging in a world of change. This unchanging is the permanent; the changing is the impermanent. This is verified at the moment of leaving the body. If one is established in the state of the unchanging, death may come and go without notice. The fundamental miracle of being is consciousness. It appears to be different than matter, but in truth it is not. Consciousness and matter are the same.

Particle physicists have been searching to identify the fundamental particle of matter. They have discovered that theses fuzzy little fast moving quanta are not particulate but are energetic: waves of energy. Energy wave quanta have, in the last few years, been shown to have two curious properties, transcendence and non-locality. An electron goes transcendent when it leaves one orbit of a nucleus and takes up residence in the next inner orbit, emitting a photon. The electron does not travel from one orbit to another. It blinks out of one orbit and reappears instantaneously in the other. Energy is transcendent.

The second quality is that of non-locality. When two related particles are emitted from an event in opposite directions; if the polarity of one particle is reversed, the polarity of the other particle reverses spontaneously and instantaneously. No signal is transmitted from one to the other, as that would violate the velocity limit of light propagation. The simultaneous polarity balance is not action at a distance, therefore is non-local. The physics of this is seen in the Proof of Bell's Theorem.

Transcendence and non-locality are characteristic of consciousness. It is unlikely that phenomena that express transcendence and non-locality are not consciousness. Thus, primacy of consciousness is established in the creation of time, space and dimension. Consciousness, the foundation of energy, also perceives the illusion of apparent difference. It is consciousness also that knows its unity; sees itself everywhere.

Consciousness is self-luminous; it is that which illumines what is. Consciousness also expresses as the power to know itself. The power is not separate or different from the light. Awareness itself is the light of the conscious universe.

If we are a seeker after Truth, at some point we will come to find Truth in our own experience. We ask: *What is it that is true, without any doubt, and is verifiable in experience?* If our blade of discrimination is sharp, we rule out everything imaginary, conceptual, inferential and illusory. In short, whatever the mind can think—is not it.

With the mind no longer a player in this quest, what does that leave us with? In the blissful stillness arises self-luminous sensory awareness of being. Nothing more. This is it. Final Truth.

Everything else we ever thought might be real or true is unverifiable as separate from our sensory awareness. In the final analysis, all else is imaginary, conceptual, inferential and illusory. Even objective reality! Is this a pen I hold in my hand? The word "pen" is a mentation that arises in consciousness and writes not. Likewise, "hand" does not feel but arises and resorbs back into consciousness.

As we lose interest in the ephemeral illusion we bring our focus to the content of this simple awareness of being. Content of awareness does not mean just witnessing sensory perception, but opening to and being filled with the rapture of eternal unbounded consciousness: our true nature.

This Truth is eternal and unchanging. Therefore in discriminating what is true and what is not we can rule out anything that was created and will, in time, be dispersed. Both physical objects and mental imaginings qualify as not the Truth. What always remains the same, was not created and shall never pass away, is the conscious ground-state of all that is.

This conscious spirit manifests as all that appears within the self-luminous awareness through its myriad pairs of eyes in infinite variety of form. The Self, seeking itself, hides within itself and is revealed through turning within to see that which is looking.

### Beyond the Beyond

*Dammit, woman! That hurt!* The deadly penicillin injection hits a tight knot in the muscle that the body knows is the last gesture of resistance before giving up to the insidious invader.

The crusty night nurse regards me with a practiced dispassion: *Just pull up your pajamas, roll over, and go to sleep. I don't want any more trouble from you."* She ambles back to her station in the otherwise unstaffed college infirmary.

I notice that something within me has become suddenly still and quiet. Has my heart stopped beating? I put my hand on my chest—nothing. I reach for the radial pulse with my other hand—nothing. Little sparkles of light dance before me as my vision begins to dim.

*Dave!* I call out to the other guy on the ward who lives on my floor in the dorm.

Darkness sweeps in.

There is a sudden rush of expansion into boundaryless awareness. I feel utter serenity infused with radiant joy. There is perfect stillness; no thoughts, no memories. In the rapturous state free from the limitations of time and space, beyond the body and the mind, I have no memory of ever having been other than **This.**

*The Buddhists know about this state. They chant:*
*Gaté, gaté, paragaté, parasamgaté. Bodhi swaha!*
*Gone, gone, utterly gone, gone without recall. O freedom!*

Gone without recall? Gone beyond remembering ever having been? O freedom! It is true!

In this vast and blissful stillness there is now movement. I am drawn toward a tunnel ringed in blue radiance. Into the tunnel through no volition of my own, I continue on around the curve in the tunnel until I see a dot of white light that grows larger as if approaching it.

Maharaj Jagat Singh writes:

"As the Soul hears the sound of the Bell and the Conch, it begins to drop off its impurities. The Soul then travels up rapidly, and flashes of the distant Light begin to come into view. Connecting the two regions is an oblique passage, called the Curved Tunnel. Only after crossing this tunnel, does the Soul reach the realm of the Creator. Here the attributes of the mind drop off and the Soul ascends alone. Once it reaches its Home, it merges in it thereby setting the Soul free." * © Maharaj Sardar Bahadur Jagat Singh Ji, <u>The Science of the Soul</u>. Radha Soami Satsang Beas. Punjab, India, p. 20.1959.

(Okay, so how did he know that the tunnel is curved? Around to the left, as I recall.)

Falling into the white light I am somehow jerked back through the tunnel and eventually enclosed into the body. The precious fullness of bliss and peace is juxtaposed in the limitations of a body thumping wildly from the epinephrine injected into my heart. The rapture is gone. I am very angry at coming back.

The Sufi Master, Hazrat Inayat Khan, gives us this teaching: "Die before death." The message here is to become established in the joyous tranquility of the inner Self so that when the body suddenly drops away we will not be distracted by attachments to the world. In this way, the Soul will complete its journey home. All of yoga is preparation for the last moment before, and the first moment after, leaving the body.

Next time I will be ready.

No fear; there is only the equipoise of the Indweller.

*Careful What You Ask For*

It is likely that a fundamental determinant of destiny is our unspent *karma;* and that probably doesn't require much further discussion; except to say that we created it, and it eventually comes back to us.

The other determinant is the power of our desires. Last night at the ashram I was having a cup of tea with a teacher of one of the meditation courses, and our conversation turned to the power of longing in determining the path of our spiritual evolution. The greater the longing, the quicker the progress. So here we see that in some measure we create our future. There is a saying in mysticism: *Careful what you ask for.* This caution implies that we will get what we ask for, and it may come when we don't want it any more, so think carefully before wishing for something.

A Sufi master once said: *You get two things in life; that which you love and that which you hate.* This broadens destiny to include whatever it is in your mind that you think of with frequency and intensity. This view is supported by the notion in yoga that whatever thoughts you are holding in your mind when you leave your body will determine content and conditions in the next incarnation. So, the finished yogi strives to purify the mind of attraction and aversion with the attention on the inner bliss, thus at the moment of release the yogi merges with the Absolute rather than coming back for another round on the wheel of *karma.* According to this, we get what we ask for in this lifetime and also in future incarnations. The key factor here is the duration and intensity with which we hold these thoughts.

So it appears that destiny is partly ordained by *karma* and partly determined by the desires of our mind. All the more reason to meditate and purify our minds of idle attachments and aversions to focus on attainments that will bring us liberation for eternity, rather than pleasure for the moment.

Another issue here relates to Guru Omkarnath remark about destiny; he said: *The book is already written, our job is to turn the pages.* Well, who is it that writes the book? Is it some God person who sits around and writes down what is to happen in our lives?

Or is it that the universe is conscious and we are holographically imbedded in a dynamic and alive process of ebb and flow of action and reaction, where *we* are the creator; and the universe forms out of itself the events and circumstances created by persistency of our creative desires? I think we are the creator as well as the player in this cosmic drama.

# Where Does It All End?

Purpose
This piece is somewhat about *karma* and reincarnation. In considering where it all will end, it would be good to look at where it all began. All that is known is that Universal Consciousness was the First Cause. It did not come into existence nor shall it ever cease to exist. There was nothing before it and nothing could remain after it. Universal Consciousness, the Self, is both the creator and the creation. As self-conscious creatures of this creation, we cycle in and out of bodies creating and burning *karma* until we figure out who we really are, what we are supposed to be doing here, and how to end these cycles of suffering. Swami Muktananda gives us great clarity about this:

> *The purpose of human life is to get knowledge of the Self. No matter how much karma a person has, when he gets knowledge of the Self, all his karmas are burned and reduced to ashes. There is no more left to reincarnate. With discrimination, knowledge, and meditation, a person should try to know his own Self.*

This is pretty amazing; all our *karmas* are burned away just by knowing the Self. Is this really true or did he just make this up?

Along with knowing the Self, the thought-free awareness of pure consciousness, *karma* and reincarnation are at the heart of mystical philosophy. This requires an abiding faith that the Universe is a conscious intelligence that is just and compassionate. Justice is assured through meditation, grace appears to burn away the *karma*, releasing the seeker from rebirth. But again, how can we be assured of the veracity of these concepts?

We can turn to the most authenticated reference for these matters: the Upanishads. These writings have been revered by great masters for thousands of years. The noted philosopher, Arthur Schopenhauer said: *In the whole world there is no study so beneficial and elevating as that of the Upanishads. It has been the solace of my life and will be the solace of my death.*

Let us sample some of the writings on the topic of the *karma* of a knower of the Self.

The Kena Upanishad says simply:

*Blessed is the man who while he yet lives realizes Brahman (the Self). The man who realizes him not, suffers his greatest loss. When they depart this life, the wise, who have realized Brahman as the Self in all beings, become immortal.*

In the <u>Katha Upanishad</u>, Lord Yama teaches Nachiketa:

*Soundless, formless, intangible, undying, tasteless, odorless, eternal, without beginning, without end, immutable, beyond nature, is the Self. Knowing him as such, one is freed from death.*

Similarly, the Mundaka Upanishad tells us:

*He who, brooding upon sense objects, comes to yearn for them, is born here and there, again and again, driven by his desire. But he who has realized the Self, and thus satisfied all hunger, attains to liberation even in this life.*

Very much to the point, the Swetasvatara Upanishad teaches:

*Only by knowing the Self does one conquer death. There is no other way of escaping the wheel of birth, death, and rebirth.*

## First Light

Gurumayi tells us to: *Meditate with the awareness that it is the Self that is meditating.* The Self is closer to us than we can possibly imagine. The Self is the creator; living as our own body. Consciousness is the watcher of our thoughts; It is the experiencer of our perceptions. It is the aliveness of our life. The Self is both seer and substance of the appearance. It is That which we think we are not. When we meditates in stillness consciousness only knows Itself. When thoughts arise, a temporary person is created, then goes out of existence again, once thoughts subside.

Consciousness contracts into thought, and observes silently as we come and go out of imagination.

We were right: we are what the Self is not. Consciousness is everything and we are nothing; but, being everything, The Self is both the everything and the nothing (no-thing).

Being the Self, we remember ourselves when we are quiet inside; and forget when the veil of thoughts darken our eyes. But happily we have seen the Truth; now we can never, ever forget.

## What is the Most Ancient Secret of Mysticism?

The most profound and fundamental miracle of existence is consciousness. What is there if there is no consciousness? Consciousness is omniscient, omnipresent, and omnipotent. It is all knowing; what can be known without consciousness? It is ever-present; even in deep sleep there is a little noise that awakens us. Who was listening? Consciousness is all-powerful; consciousness is the groundstate of our intelligence.

It was Saint Francis who made the brilliant observation: *That which you are looking for is That which is looking.* But the Self, or consciousness, *is* knowable. It is through meditation on the awareness of just being that we become conscious of consciousness. This is the profound state of mystical union that all seekers strive to attain. This is liberation, this is transcendence, this is the enlightened state.

It is consciousness that sees through our eyes, and feels the warmth of the sun. It is consciousness that knows the thoughts of our mind. To know the Self is simply to awaken to the radiant illumination of inner stillness that reveals pure consciousness itself.

The fundamental wisdom in mysticism is that the Self is the unseen Seer seeing out of our eyes. It is mysterious how this unseen Seer came to take up residence in this body. After all, it is not the body that sees, it is the conscious indweller that reads the senses.

Like the sun, the Seer illuminates all that is before it. Darkness only arises when something obscures the light of the sun. Similarly, the darkness of ignorance only arises when the mind (ego) obscures the self-luminous Seer. Thoughts in the mind distract the Seer from its natural state of immersion in the blissful contentment of just being.

When faced with an insoluble mystery, the mind often resorts to logic to escape the cognitive dissonance of the perplexity. We prefer the comfort of deduction to the ambiguity of mystery even if the deduction runs counter to our experience.

Whatever arises in the mind is imaginary: the word water does not quench the thirst, the thought of light does not cause the darkness to recede. In our quest, only the witness of the mind knows Truth, seeing things just as they are.

The purpose of breathing-in the stillness is to become the witness. It is the conscious Self that sees through our eyes, knows our thoughts and feels what is in our hearts. Similarly, it is through the inner stillness that we come to know the Self.

In the stillness of meditation the knower is revealed. The seer is seen. In the stillness, the mind is purified of the veil that obscures the perfection within.

The conscious indweller that is the Self, is eternal. Our consciousness is not only deathless, it is without sorrow, without hunger or thirst, without craving (desire); it is ever joyful, utterly at peace and everflowing in love. We know the fullness of this presence in the inner stillness beyond the mind. We are, in our hearts, this divine, serene and loving Spirit.

Ahh, the Ocean of Bliss; the very wellspring of divine love.
Eternal, yet lost in time...
All pervasive, yet hidden from sight...
All powerful, yet fragile in our grasp...
All knowing, yet forgotten...
Infinite, yet nothing (no-thing)...
Blissful, yet distracted to sorrow...
Mysterious to the mind, yet revealed in the heart...
Ahh, the Ocean of Bliss:
We discover what was never lost,
return to where we never left.

In this utter serenity and total awareness is the state that transcends and survives the death of the body, and it is ours while still in the body.

In attaining this thought-free equanimity, we see the true nature of reality. We know who we are for the first time. We are awakened; no longer sleeping in our mind. This is a sweet and entertaining dream, but it is better when we wake up. Everything will be different and everything will be the same.

[from a letter to Cheryl]

You asked how does one love another who is persistently unlovable. Trying to love someone else only perpetuates the fundamental ignorance of our view of the world—that there is anyone else. So what do we do about that person who causes us to simmer inside? The only thing I have found that works is to become so absorbed in the inner bliss that when we look out from within we are so immersed in the fountain of love that arises naturally from the heart, that the appearance is simply entertainment, no matter how pleasurable or painful it might be. When we see, we see the light of our own consciousness; when we feel, we feel the fullness of our own heart. This takes utter dedication to purification of the mind so that we can see deeply into the stillness and surrender to the sweetness that is our own being. In short; meditation.

As we both know, this doesn't come naturally, nor are we entrained to the practice and experience by our society to merge back into the ocean of love from which we emerged. Once we touch that inner stillness, we must go back again, and again, and again. Through this practice we gradually empty out the conditioning of the mind to make way for the flood of joy that forever washes our perceptions pure of any incoming dissonance.

We are so full of our own love we can choose to be filled by it, rather than absorb the poisons from outside the imaginary boundary with someone else. Gurumayi said once, I *choose this state every moment.*

Let's take a critical look at loving another. Imagine that you love someone—you embrace her or him—where does the love come from? Does it come from that person or does it arise within your own heart? Can you really give love to someone else? Can another give love to you? What is your real experience of this?

Ultimately, we don't have to love anyone else, we only have to allow the fullness of the inner bliss to fill our awareness through persistence in meditation. If love truly is *motiveless tenderness of the heart,* we just remain self-absorbed in that tenderness as the witness to the appearance. Out there, it just is what it is.

You want to know,

"Or does liberation bring a feeling of love toward all that is free of the emotions attached to form?"

Yes; but the love is not directed at others; love is an undirected presence.

"How can I get there quick?"

In immediate situations where feelings come up that are other than loving, I take refuge in the *mantra*. When I feel the burning, I go immediately to *Om Namah Shivaya* to absorb the mind and emotions until I'm back in balance. Usually it doesn't take long. In the private stillness of meditation the *mantra* becomes associated with the deep bliss of the Self. Out in the world also, mentally repeating the *mantra* will take us to the associated place of the compassionate steady state.

## What Do You Want From Meditation?

Trick question!

Wanting anything disturbs meditation; even wanting peaceful meditation is a desire, and disturbs meditation. We sit for meditation to find peace. This is also our laboratory where we observe the mind and determine the problems and solutions of bringing the mind to peace. First we observe that our mind is constantly stirring the drama of wanting something we don't have, having something we don't want, and wanting someone or something to be different. This is living in a perfect storm of endless desires. It is no wonder that we want meditation to bring us peace.

The first thing the mind discovers is that it must step aside for peacefulness to awaken. This is a shock to the ego and it resists vigorously. Progress is gradual but we begin getting glimpses of the sweetness that arises spontaneously. Over time we learn that desires are the primary disturbance of our inner peace. We are deeply conditioned to desire everything from the world, but we eventually learn that these desires only brings suffering. On this path of yoga and meditation we see the tendency to turn inward as we progress in our sadhana. Turning inward we discover that the happiness we wanted from the world is already present in the stillness of just being. Amazing.

From here, all there is to do is deepen in the stillness, the fullness of the emptiness. In this contented serenity, we take the bliss of the Self out into the world.

*When the mind sheds its desires,*
*it finds the sweetness of peace and bliss.*
~Gurumayi

## Is Anything Real?

Studying the literature of *Vedanta* (Yoga Philosophy) we see repeated references to the notion that the world is unreal, or illusory (*maya*). This is crazy. I know in my own experience that the solid objects around me are real, and no amount of philosophy will convince me otherwise. So what's going on here; is this world really real or not?

To make any progress at all on this perplexity let's look at where this notion of *maya* came from. The great *rishis* who gave us these concepts did so in a different language, *Sanskrit*. Many of these great works have fortunately been translated into English. It is here in the translation that we can look and see what the original vision was in describing domains of universal consciousness and living in the world.

Fundamentally we see clearly that existence includes the changing and the unchanging, the ephemeral and the eternal. The ephemeral is the world of nature that we see around us. It is certainly intuitive to know that everything changes over time; we all see this happening. Then, what is the eternal unchanging, if everything changes? The *watcher* of the changing never changes. Consciousness performs no action, has no thought or memory; it is simply the light of awareness by which we know everything. It has no form, is in no place, was not created, and cannot be changed or destroyed. Consciousness is the foundation and substance of the universe. Nothing came before,

118

and nothing comes after. The *rishis*, observing these outer and inner phenomena say that everything is *sat* (existence) or *asat* (non-existent). *Sat* is also the Sanskrit root for *satya*, truth. Thus existence is true, and non-existence is untrue.

Whatever arises in the mind is imaginary and is always changing. These mental perspectives vary between individuals so there is really no verifiable consistency; which makes the mind *asat*: not true. But consciousness, the impartial observer, sees things just as they are; this is *sat*, true. Unfortunately, *sat* and *asat* have been translated as real and unreal. It would have been more accurate to use the English words of unchanging and changing to imply *sat* and *asat*.

Now we know that, yes, the world exists and is real, even though it is changing. But whatever we think about it is the *maya*, illusion, the unreal. We make up this ego drama of our life and live in it as if it were real, until we sit quietly and touch the stillness. In the stillness we become the watcher, we see things just as they are. This is truth, *satya*. *Sadhana* is the process of purifying the mind and living as the watcher.

There is a paradox here; the mind knows about this sublime concept of *sat* and *asat*, but knowing about it, is not it. Only when the mind is still do we have the experience of self-aware consciousness, the Self that is real, true, and unchanging. The good news is that the mind learns about stillness in the experience of meditation, and becomes more content within the quiet. The ego surrenders to the bliss of transcendence. We find the balance where the mind is allowed to do what it is good for (logic, navigation, etc.), with the default state of seeing things just as the are.

## Vairagya

There are two fundamentals on this path that are required for liberation. The first is *viveka*; distinguishing consciousness (the perceiver) from the mind (an object of perception). Second is *vairagya*; commonly defined as non-attachment, or dispassion.

If we do not develop these two sensitivities, we remain ignorant of the Self (*avidya*), our truest identity. Without *vairagya*, there is no peace.

Let us look carefully at *vairagya*. Right understanding will show us what it is, and right action will integrate the concept into our behavior. There is more resistance to non-attachment in the west because of our powerful cultural conditioning of ownership and control. Look at how deeply this conditioning is rooted even in our normal thinking. Most of our thought traffic is about wanting something we don't have, having something we don't want, or wanting something or someone to be different than they are. The tentacles of desire and discontent reach deeply into our relationship with our self, our family, and our culture.

Beginning this path we find it incomprehensible to not be attached to our family, our things, and our opinions. But this is a path of turning inward so that we actually see and feel the inner effects of our thoughts and actions. Through the practice of meditation we bring the mind to stillness. In the contentment of observing thoughts and actions, we discover that obsessing over attachment and control does not bring us peace. Here we have to choose: do we continue the self-destructive clinging of expectation, or do we become the watcher and just follow *dharma*?

*Vairagya* does not mean that we do not care, or no longer feel compassion. Living with mindfulness is simply allowing everything to be just as it is. Relationship *dharma* includes caring and compassion, but not the destructive disharmony of attachment. Letting go of this insidious darkness brings inner (and outer) peace and happiness.

Historically we recognize the Buddha's iconic teaching: *The cause of suffering is craving.* Every little desire that creeps into our thoughts create disappointment and resentment. Now we have the choice of disturbance, or peacefulness. No doubt the mind will offer myriad justifications to keep immersion in the drama, but it's just the ego needing attention. This is now optional.

*ATTENTION!*

Where is the primary focus of your attention as you go through your day? Isn't it in the mind? Don't we depend on the mind to identify objects in appearance, to regurgitate opinions about the objects, to determine what actions are appropriate regarding the appearance, and to determine what is next in our processing of all this information and action? These are all useful functions of the mind, but we also know that the mind is in the way of spiritual development, direct knowing, truth, and wisdom. So what has gone wrong, where did we miss something? Can we live without the mind? How do we resolve this confusion?

The mind is the platform for memories and conditioning, and a conduit for sensory information to and from consciousness. Through the practice of meditation we can take control of this conduit of information, allowing more or less to pass through depending on our needs at the time. When consciousness takes the form of the mind, it cannot be Self-aware. To enable Self-awareness we must shift our attention away from the mind, to the breath, the mantra, or the stillness. This is the skill we must develop in meditation, refocusing our attention away from the selfishness of the ego, to the serenity and contentment of the thought-free Self.

Much is attained in this skill of refocusing attention to the stillness. The mind is disciplined to work when it is useful and to be still at other times. In this stillness we know our Self for the first time; we find the peace and bliss of just being, and we illumine in our experience pure consciousness that is boundaryless and eternal. This is who we are.

The mind does not surrender easily and it's a constant struggle to quiet the mind and live as the Peaceful Presence. What can we do? What practice is there to ease this transition?

Once we know our essential identity as consciousness, we can then dis-identify with the mind and the senses. We isolate the mind by discriminating it from consciousness, then lose interest in the mind. We isolate the senses by identifying perception as *abhasa*, then lose interest in perceptions that arise. This requires much practice, but if this is your path, it is not a burden.

Once we attain mastery over mind and senses, we come to the process of surrender. Who surrenders, and what is surrendered? The fact is that we are not the body, mind, or senses; we have just been conditioned to believe this. Through meditation we awaken to glimpse our true nature. Practicing the inner stillness over a long period of time naturally brings us to become the stillness. This is surrender, gradually becoming who we have always been. We simply turn away from what is not us, shining as the blissful Self. Forever.

## Breaking Up Is Hard To Do

We can look back on our broken relationships and wonder why it was so painful for so long. What is it about relationships that makes it so hard to let go when it is over? What can we do to mitigate our disappointment and anger when this precious bond falls apart?

It seems so natural to form attachment to those who have drawn close to us; how can we not be attached to one we care so much for?

On this path of yoga and meditation we find inner peace as relief from the outer pain. Naturally the first teaching we encounter on this path is the injunction to let go all attachments. This is where we start if we truly want peace in our life. Certainly it is clear that if we have no attachment we would abound in serenity; but how do we live in the world with no attachment?

First, let's look critically at attachment and see what the problem is. Attachment is an emotional dependence on someone or some thing outside us to make us happy. We make up the expectation that this person will always love us and behave the way we expect. Really, what are the possibilities that this will work? Expectation is the poison in relationships. What to do?

Coming to yoga and meditation is a turning within. We practice sitting quietly, opening the inner eye, and find sweetness and well-being, a steady state just behind the mind. This is a gradual revelation, but in time we come to live as the peaceful presence. In this we are at peace with our surroundings and at peace with the world. We are full and happy no matter what the world brings us or takes away. Everything comes to us, and everything leaves us. We are the contented observer of things and people coming and going.

It's not that we don't care, it's that we see things just as they are and don't need to control everything. It is our dharma to share affection and caring in the family. In that, we fulfill all our relationships. There is no need for expectation or attachment. When we are free of fearful clutching and clinging, all those you touch will experience a new lightness. What a relief.

It is easy to say, *just let go*; but more thinking about it just thickens the quicksand. We must put in the time to bring stillness to the drunken monkey chattering in our head. Sit quietly every day, refocus your awareness to the breath or mantra. Have no expectations of your state while sitting, just sit. Then again tomorrow; then again. We are like a capacitor, accumulating bliss as we sit in meditation. The sublime serenity does indeed accumulate over time, and ultimately we feel happy and content in every moment.

### MEDITATION: True Love

What is it that *true love* has in common with *meditation*? And how is true love different than our common concept of love? We begin with meditation, sitting quietly to touch the stillness. What we find when we first sit is a cacophony of thoughts and feelings that spontaneously arise when we close our eyes. It is intimidating to hope for quiet in the midst of the noise. At this point it is critical to begin the practice of focusing on a single thing; the breath, the mantra. It is in this focused attention that the storm of thoughts and feelings begin to subside. This is a gradual process that works best if we sit quietly every day.

One reason we must do this practice is because the mind is not accustomed to stillness. We need to take the myriad thoughts and reduce them down to one thing. Once we can focus on just one thing; the next step is focusing on just the stillness. This is not easy, but it does arise naturally with persistence in practice. Be patient.

The other reason for the practice is that we must separate the conscious observer from the contents of the mind. Consciousness is the watcher; the mind is simply a conduit of sensory information. Thus we create a separation between unchanging consciousness (the Self) and the ever-changing mind.

The purpose of meditation is to still the mind; this brings the steady state. But why do we even want the stillness? In the emptiness (*shunya*) we begin to explore the experience of our inward turning awareness. At first it is just empty. In time we begin to experience the fullness of serenity, and moments of sweetness that arise spontaneously. This is our true nature. This is the love that is ourself (our Self). Immersion in the fullness of the stillness brings us happiness and contentment no matter what happens in the changing world. The steadiness of true love sustains us.

A great saint tells us that, *Love is motiveless tenderness of the heart. Motiveless* means no expectation. *Tenderness* means tender all the time. Does this characterize your love relationships? Think about this! Normally we think of love as affection and dependency with the expectation that the pleasure will last. When the pleasure fades, do we fall out of love? Through the practice of meditation, the inner love fulfills us while outer loves come and go.

The Siddha Master, Gurumayi Chidvilasananda tells us, *Once the fountain of love is unlocked in our hearts, we see the magnificence of our existence. With that love we turn the world into a paradise.* This is the inner love that develops as we become established in the inner sweetness of just being. If this is what we want, then it is the longing that powers our path of awakening.

# The Mystery of Consciousness

## What Is The True Nature Of Consciousness?

This question is asked by only a few, and of those, few come to know some answer beyond opinion, and verifiable in experience. This is not so surprising; consciousness cannot be objectified, because it is ever the subject. It is real yet neither concrete nor abstract. We cannot be without it, but if it were gone, we would not miss it. We cannot see it because it is the seer. It being the knower, can it be known? Consciousness does not act nor can it be acted upon. It is unitary (non-relational) because there is no other subject. Consciousness has no qualities but possesses a quality-less quality that can only be known when the mind is still and awareness becomes simply the observer.

Consciousness is... so it has being; and this beingness has its own nature. Fundamentally it is the principle of illumination by which all else is known and has the power to know itself. Consciousness is the fundamental ground-state of all being and knowing. Understanding this as a concept is simple, knowing the knower is a bit more challenging.

## Is Consciousness Universal Or Only Local?

Our common experience of being conscious is indeed a local event. However we have all had intuitions about things at a distance or outside of time that can best be explained if we think of consciousness as a field, unlimited by time or space. There is good evidence that we can know events and even communicate with others not in our immediate time and place—not often, to be sure; but it happens.

## Why Hasn't Science Investigated Consciousness?

Consciousness has no mass or volume, therefore cannot be sampled, measured, analyzed, dissected, qualitated or quantitated. It is a field with no charge, polarity, density or effect. It is a state that cannot be observed, created or destroyed. In short: to science, consciousness is a mystery. One science writer called it, "The ghost in the machine."

The field of psychology is more a study of the mind than an inquiry into the nature of consciousness. These are two very different things. Consciousness is the observer of the mind so does not fall under the purview of psychology.

Philosophy perhaps comes a little closer, but still, philosophy is more concerned with epistemology (ways of knowing) rather than discerning the knower.

Mysticism, however, **is** the science of consciousness. There is no higher goal in mysticism than to embrace the thought-free conscious self-awareness that reveals the nectar of equipoise and ecstasy inherent in pure consciousness. This mystical union hides behind such rubrics as Buddha Nature, Zen Mind, Brahman, Tao, Yahweh, etc. This is a sweeping conjecture, but consciousness is immutable and eternal, all knowing and ever-present.

## Where Does Consciousness Come From? ...And Go To?

All things that are compounded will eventually be dispersed. It appears that consciousness is not compounded from other things, so it may not readily disperse. All that exists is either created or was always in existence. We all know that physics generally holds that the material universe formed from an unknowable event 14 billion years ago that gave birth to leptons (electrons, etc.), hadrons (quarks -> protons, neutrons), bosons (photons, etc.) as well as various forces from which our common objects are made. The seminal event is said to be unknowable because of what some call Planck's Wall; a short period of time(?) after the big bang in which the state of the soon-to-be universe did not follow the rules of quantum physics. None of this addresses the issue of consciousness as it seems not to have been formed with the rest of the known universe. Nor is there evidence that it formed since then.

In the absence of other information we might speculate that consciousness has always existed and may continue to exist, independent of sentient creatures to address it locally. I know, this is hard to imagine.

One might think of consciousness as an emergent property of life but it is difficult to draw the line between sentient and non-sentient life. Science is unable to show this.

## Does Consciousness Survive The Death Of The Body?

There is much heat and little light about this question. There are many consistent reports about consciousness continuing after all clinical signs of life cease. So all those who have not had this experience are left with only their opinions as to whether death of the body is final. The author has had the memorable experience of an excellent and expanded awareness for some time beyond clinical death after total cardiopulmonary collapse. My experience says that consciousness does continue.... For how long, I couldn't say; as time and space seemed not relevant to the state. There is a boundary, or event horizon, beyond which the laws of quantum mechanics do not apply; sort of a Planckian Epoch.

## Can inert matter be conscious?

Common sense would tell you that this could not be. However....

In the 1930s Einstein (and Podolsky and Rosen) refuted Heisenburg's Uncertainty Principle that said, in part, that quantum events must occur locally within the space-time continuum. In the1980s John Bell and Alain Aspect proved Einstein right. In what is called the proof of Bell's Theorem, two photons from the valence electron of a calcium ion are emitted with opposite polarities. Using a polarization filter, Alain Aspect flipped the polarity of one of the photons and monitored the paired photon. At the same instant the paired photon spontaneously flipped its polarity. How did it know to do that? And how did one photon communicate with its partner in no elapsed time? Physicists call this a "non-local" effect. Ten years later, four different physicists (Capra, Zukav, Goswami and Herbert) published books on this event and suggested that consciousness is the universal (non-local, transcendent) field that is not bound to the space-time continuum. They further suggest that consciousness is the ground-state from which all energy and matter arise, so that ultimately all matter and energy is not different than consciousness itself. This is how the paired electrons know to maintain coherent polarity: they are simply vectors of consciousness itself.

Now; can inert matter be conscious? How can it not be conscious? That is its nature!

## When We Sleep Are We Still Conscious?

The mind is asleep, consciousness, the witness, is awake. While you are sleeping perhaps a noise awakens you. Who was listening to the noise?

## Is Consciousness The Same As, Or Different From The Mind?

The mind is local to the brain but consciousness is non-local. When the brain dies, the mind dies; but consciousness, the universal field, remains. It might be useful to think of the mind as a contraction of consciousness. The mind is a complex instrument of perception that includes ego, memory and rationality. In the intimate relationship between consciousness and the mind, consciousness is the perceiver, the mind is the instrument of perceiving. Importantly, consciousness can know the mind but the mind cannot know consciousness.

## The Deification Of Consciousness

Western physics is not the first or only system to assert the universality of consciousness. This has been recognized since antiquity in the east. We find references to it in the most ancient writings known to humankind, primarily in the Indus Valley and the mountain regions of northern India and Kashmir. The science of knowing the knower has generally not been common knowledge in any culture over time but has remained esoteric, the knowledge being passed down from teacher to student through the ages. Cultures change but the core teachings about the nature and experience of pure consciousness have remained consistent. Even today the core teachings of mysticism are consistent across cultures.

It is this experience gained through the practice of meditation upon the pure awareness of being that is at the core of the esoteric teachings. Adepts of this practice are known as mystics and the body of literature that has built up over the millennia is the arcana of mysticism.

Because of the profundity of equanimity and inspiration reached in the meditative state, great reverence is given both to the experience and to the masters of the state. In ancient times this mastery was widely celebrated in the eastern cultures, and is to this day.

The focus on the pure experience of consciousness through meditative discipline is the primal root of religious micro-culture. History has shown that over time, unless there continues to be a lineage of enlightened teachers, the religion will fall into political hierarchy and lose the spiritual essence of the original imperative. Images are created as a focus for devotion when the pure inner light no longer shines.

# Song of the Buddha

I remember when I was a child and they called me the Prince Gautama. Having no brothers or sisters to play with I was immersed in an adult world; mother was my most constant companion. Father watched over me with keen interest, but from a little distance. The servants were ever-attentive making life on the estate full to overflowing with all I could think to need. Little did I know that this was a planned indulgence to distract me from a destiny foretold by the seers.

The whole of my childhood was spent in play and in learning the stories from the Ramayana and Mahabharata. As I grew older I became a little restless and wanted to know more of the world, even though all my needs were met right here on the estate.

When I came of age my father arranged my marriage. My bride was quite lovely and in time I became absorbed in my new life as householder. As the seasons came around again I became a father; my son shone like the moon. He too, surely, would be a prince among men.

But once again the longing reappeared to see life outside the estate. One day while my father was away on a journey, my companion Govinda, close like a brother, came to me and asked me to accompany him on a visit into town. I quickly accepted. Through the gates we rode, then out into the countryside — how beautiful and open, but not as well manicured as the orchards of the estate.

As we approached the town I spied a wretched dried-up creature begging alms. To Govinda I said, "*What is that?*"

"Just a beggar" he said.

"Can't we help him?"

"There is nothing to be done." replied he.

We also passed by a funeral procession, then into town. More beggars, some lame; garbage in heaps; unhappiness, pain and deprivation.

"Sri Ram! Why this suffering?"

And my companion could only say; "This is the way it is, there is no help for it."

I became crazed by the torment of human suffering; I must find out why; I must do something about it. I must come to understand this pity of human existence.

Back at the estate the chilling specter haunted me day and night. I became obsessed to find the answer.

I arose early in the morning, went to my wife and told her what I must do. I kissed my sleeping son and departed my father's estate.

Taking the road to the forest I chanced upon three wandering sadhus and told them of my search, and they guided me to a small camp of holy men staying by the river. I asked many of them for the answers to my questions. Some told me the same as Govinda; "*There is no help for it.*" Others just looked at me and said nothing.

Since the wise men didn't know, it was clear that I must find out for myself. Therefore I resolved to sit in contemplation until I was able to divine the "why" and "what to do" of suffering, and to find a Truth that would not decay.

For a long time I sat, hardly moving. The old sage who never spoke brought me water from time to time, and occasional fruit. After 20 seasons of straining to the breaking point for the answers I sought, I could find no reason for the suffering and decay. Finally I had to give up. I had failed. No longer could I continue this suffering in the name of suffering. The despair of failure collapsed my mind into nothingness.

For a long time I rested in the stillness; the passion of my desire for understanding was broken. In this tranquility I realized that my suffering had ceased and joy was welling up in my heart. And from the depths within, my Soul pleaded to be released from the limitation of the mind.

"*Is this the answer to suffering?*" I thought again of the pain of suffering, and I felt again the depth of perfect peace, free from desire.

For 49 more days sitting by the river I experienced the Truth that transcended decay, and surrendered to my Soul that expanded through the vastness of the Universe. I savored the sweetness of new understanding; that the nature of being is pure awareness, the light of intelligence, and the bliss of contentment.

Such great compassion arose for the plight of those enchanted by craving for the ephemeral that brings only grief and another round on the wheel of karma. Surely the travail for the many continues because such a one has never walked among them who is free from the tyranny of the mind and the clutching of the heart. If this be the case then the end has come to my solitude in the forest.

I must go now and hold the lamp for those who seek the light, to remind those who have forgotten who they are, and teach those who would exchange despair for eternal happiness.

First I will rejoin five of my fellow seekers who endured with me the years of austerities while in search of the Eternal amidst the mysteries of the ephemeral. They departed for a city to the south; a center of spiritual erudition. I will follow them along the two weeks travel from Bodhgaya to Varanasi. There is time to arrive before the beginning of the monsoons, a time when a traveler must find shelter against the torrents of renewal.

These days of travel will be time to reflect upon the knowledge and experiences that arose not of the mind but as illuminations of the Soul. This has not been a tautology of deduction, but a sort of remembering of self-evident truth emerging out of the stillness of just sitting.

The dust of the road mixes with the company of merchants, pilgrims, and other travelers to form the ever-changing scene playing in the background. The sublime rapture of pure being, unmolested by the discontent of the mind or hunger of the senses, forms the fullness of the inner presence. I feel a radiance within me that reaches out in recognition of all those who pass. They are, in fact, my own Self looking out through so many eyes. But sadly, the expressions around so many eyes tell the story of preoccupation with concerns of circumstance, memory of what is no more, and fear of what might be.

The way to Varanasi widens at the approach to the great Ganges River. A few more days along the river road and my destination will be at hand.

Varanasi announces itself in the distance with the haze of straw and dung cooking fires punctuated by plumes of smoke from the burning ghats. Many come to Varanasi to leave their body in the belief that cremation there by the Ganges will assure the soul a place in heaven.

In time I am reunited with my companions. It is to them that I first disclose the Four Noble Truths and the Eight Means of Attainment. They listen in curious respect as they notice that they are watched by the unmoving seer. The five are enveloped in the serenity that walks in these footsteps. They ask to be taught the way to Nirvana.

"You know already of the existence of suffering that is rooted in attachment and aversion. Understand that the cause of suffering is due to the craving in the mind for what does not exist, the craving of the senses for transitory pleasures, and craving in the heart for the good opinion of those who do not love themselves. Understand also that the remedy of suffering is through dispassion: indifference to the contents of the mind, transcendence of the appetites of the senses, and stilling the restlessness of the heart.

"The path leading to cessation of suffering is through the Eight Means of Attainment: right views, right aspirations, right speech, right behavior, right livelihood, right effort, right thought, and right contemplation.

"Right views are cultivated through study of the scriptures and the practice of non-attachment to the ephemeral things of the world; this is the torch to light the way. Aspire to be content in every moment, long for refuge in Buddha Nature; this shall be your guide. Right speech is found in truthfulness. Right behavior requires non-injury, non-stealing, forbearance, moderation, and restraining of the passions. Right livelihood is enjoyed wherever Buddha Dharma is followed and charity is served. Perseverance in bringing to rest the chattering of the mind is right effort. Right thoughts are free from the past, unafraid of the future, and undisturbed by the present. Right contemplation is the silent witness to the truth of pure being, immersed in serenity, unmoved by the tides of change, and filled with joy at just breathing in and breathing out.

"Oh brothers, this revelation is not in the least intended to make you self-righteous. Even pray that no one ever notices your attainment of Nirvana. Treading this path is to free you from the bondage of ignorance, loose the chains of karma, and bring you peace."

The monks, hearing the words and feeling the presence, knew that it was true. All that is left now is to hold to the teachings. In time, they too will become the Buddha.

# Just for Fun

*The Story of Bija and Lotus Blossom*

Once upon a time long ago and far away there lived the great King Kumara in the beautiful and peaceful land of Vrindavan. Kumara was a good and wise king, fair to all his subjects and generous to those in need.

Vrindavan was lush and green with a wide and lazy river running through it. The peaceful valley where the town was located was surrounded on three sides by beautiful hills thick with trees.

Upon one of these hills in a thicket of big trees lived the monk Bija. Now Bija was no ordinary monk who just contemplated the nature of being and performed ceremonies when asked, Bija had the power of enchantment. He even lived in an enchanted house. You could tell this when trying to find your way to his little abode. Everyone in the town knew which hill he lived on, there was even a trail up the hill, but hardly anyone ever wanted to go there. Bija was a hermit of sorts and was quite different from the townspeople in that he didn't have a farm or a shop and he never came to town.

If anyone did try to follow the trail up to his house and did not have a pure heart, then the trail would wind round and round and eventually lead back to the bottom of the hill. Only the pure of heart could find their way straight to Bija's little house.

It so happened that there lived, in the beautiful and peaceful land of Vrindavan, a maiden of rare charm and loveliness. Her name was Lotus Blossom and she was a miller's daughter. She lived with her mother and father at the mill house by the river. While her father tended the mill, which ground grain from the valley into flour, Lotus Blossom and her mother wove the material to make into flour sacks. Then on market days her father would take the sacks of flour into town in a horse cart to sell or trade.

It is true that Lotus Blossom is an unusual name. When she was born, her parents saw that she was so fair of face and form that an ordinary name just wouldn't do. Most of the girls of that day had names like Surya, Urvashi and Ganga. She was of such surpassing beauty that her parents decided to name her after a flower. The Lotus is very special in that it lives in the water but the flower opens above the water and remains untouched by it. And as it proved to be in the life of the miller's daughter, she lived in the ways of the townspeople but remained untouched by the struggles and injustices of life in the world.

Lotus Blossom helped her parents in many ways as they went about the business of the mill. One of the chores she did every morning was to go down to the river and fill the water urn that she carried very gracefully upon her head. Just by coincidence Bija, the reclusive monk and sometimes advisor to the king, happened to be gathering herbs early one morning down by the river bank. As he was walking along the river gazing intently at the grasses and shrubs growing there he heard in the distance, singing. He stopped abruptly and listened. "Hmmm," he thought, "that is quite lovely; methinks I hear magic in that voice." The song finished, Bija stood still for a moment or two then hurried round the bend in the river to behold the source of the angelic refrain. He looked and there was no one there. "Well; either the angel lives close by or my grandfather (from whom he learned his sorcery) has sent a spirit to sport with me. We shall see in the sun-up of the morrow which is what."

With that he slung his sack of herbs over his shoulder and returned to his little house on the hill.

All day and into the night Bija couldn't decide which he would rather deal with; an angel with magic in her voice, or a spirit of beguilement sent from the other side.

Up before dawn and on his way to the river, Bija was ready to untangle the mystery. Surely enough as the sun was burning away the dew drops from the flower petals on the meadow, he heard the sweetly lilting voice of Lotus Blossom drawing near to him.

Quickly he hid himself in the purple shade of a great Cypress lording over the riverbank, and then he saw her…. The water urn balanced perfectly atop her head, her slender body swayed to and fro as she walked slowly and gracefully on her morning errand. Her simple homespun peasant dress lent an air of reserve to the sparkle of her byzantine eyes and her face shown pink, like alabaster in the sunrise. Bija sensed about her strength and tenderness, intelligence and simplicity, excitement and serenity.

He watched as she easily unseated the urn from atop her dark braids wound round the top of her head, and in a single motion kneeled to fill the vessel with clear cold river water recently melted from the snow of the mountains. When it was filled to the weight of her satisfaction she placed it beside her and gazed out across the river to the wooded banks on the other side. There she sat seemingly lost in reverie as she rested awhile after the walk from the mill house.

In the stillness Bija noticed he had hardly taken a breath or thought a single word as he watched in rapt attention the unfolding of this lovely scene.

"Hello Bija," Whispered a gentle voice within his mind.

"Whozzat!?" Said a startled and befuddled Bija.

Lotus Blossom turned and smiled.

Unable to fully grasp what had just happened Bija stared wide-eyed with no words coming from his open mouth. A fragment of a previous thought came to him "…methinks I hear magic in that voice."

"Oh no, this can't be." Said Bija to no one in particular.

"Would you like to walk me home?" Bija still hadn't moved…

"My name is Lotus Blossom. I live at the mill house." She arose lifting the water jar to its traveling perch.

As she slowly strode toward the Cypress and its immobilized companion, Bija adjusted his vision slightly out of focus and looked to the side of her so as to see her spirit. What he saw was a radiant light-being three times life size with golden rays issuing forth from her heart and a violet glow at the outer edges of the radiance of white light.

Thought Bija to himself, "Truly this is an angel come from heaven to bring goodness and grace upon the Earth." And again from within came a giggle, and, "Thank you."

They stood and looked at each other, both knowing everything. Their minds and hearts blended together seeing the vision of the entire universe and knowing all past, present and future. They remembered before time when they were one soul. They saw their many lifetimes, twin souls finding each other time after time. They transcended the infinite, merging into the ocean of bliss becoming one again. They saw themselves in each other's eyes; two, yet one. Separate, yet united. Different, yet the same. Mortal, yet divine.

Thus it was that Bija and Lotus Blossom were together once again, this time in the wondrous land of Vrindavan. They beheld each other like two raindrops risen from the sea, seeing in each other both themselves and the unity from which they emerged. They knew also that their souls would merge again in time and in another millennium play at the drama of separation and remembrance. Mayhaps even now they are reaching out for the heart that, in truth, is their own.

# Glossary of Terms

**Ahamkara**: Fundamental aspect of the ego that maintains the sense of individuality; the I-consciousness.

**Anava Mala**: Fundamental ignorance of one's true identity with consciousness and bliss.

**Anugraha**: Grace: The power of an awakened teacher to reveal the student's own divine nature.

**Arjuna**: A major character in the Bhagavad Gita who is taught Yoga dharma by his charioteer, Lord Krishna.

**Aum**: A spelling of OM, the Sanskrit sound symbol for the Transcendent Eternal.

**Avatar**: Incarnation of God.

**Bhagavad Gita**: Scriptural story revealing Yoga dharma.

**Bhagavatam**: Scripture of devotional Yoga.

**Brahman**: Universal Absolute. Transcendent Truth. Universal ground-state.

**Buddhi**: Discriminative aspect of the ego that sees the world relationally; I – that.

**Buddha Nature**: State of compassionate detachment. Samadhi.

**Darshan**: The company of, or blessing by, an enlightened being.

**Dharma**: Righteousness sustained through noble virtues.

**Ephemeral**: Fleeting existence or appearance in any time scale. Anything that is created and will eventually disperse; from atoms to galaxies, from thoughts to ideologies.

**Enlightenment**: To awaken to the conscious witness observing the mind and live fully in the transcendent joy and equipoise of our true nature.

**Gunas**: Qualities in nature: Sattva (pure, steady, joyous), Rajas (active, stimulating), Tamas (heavy, dense, indifferent).

**Hesychast Order**: Catholic order of monks who practice a meditation of inner stillness.

**Hrdaya:** The heart center, seat of consciousness.

**Iccha Shakti:** The power of will.

**Jiva:** The empirical self; conscious indweller of the host body. Local address of the Universal Absolute.

**Jnana:** Knowledge, wisdom, comprehension.

**Jnana Yoga:** The yoga of spiritual wisdom.

**Karma:** Consequential thread of willful actions performed with expectation of the outcome. An action performed with no attachment to outcome incurs no karma. Beneficence with motive brings eventual beneficial karma. Intentional harmful action bring similar consequences to the doer in this lifetime or another.

**Karma Mala:** Mistaken identity that the separate ego is the doer of action. Upon awakening, the jiva realizes that the Universal Self is the doer of all action.

**Kashmir Shaivism:** Non-dual school of Tantra philosophy.

**Khechari Mudra:** Refined understanding that the yogi is merged in consciousness that moves in all beings.

**Kirtan:** Devotional singing or chanting the name of God.

**Kriya Shakti:** The power of action. One of the three powers of Consciousness; the other two being Icca (will), and Jnana (knowledge). The action frequently associated with this power of Consciousness, is thought.

**Kundalini Shakti:** The conscious spiritual energy that commonly lies dormant in the muladhara chakra at the base of the spine. Once awakened, bliss breaks out in the heart chakra.

When the kundalini reaches the sahasrara (crown chakra), spiritual maturity is complete (samadhi).

**Maha Maya:** The divine power of obscuration. Consciousness hides from itself by raising a veil of thoughts across awareness. The veil is drawn back in the stillness of meditation.

**Mala:** Constriction of transcendent consciousness. The three malas are anava (ignorance of the true Self), mayiya (illusion of separation) and karma (actions that create karmic debt).

**Manas**: The recording faculty of the mind that receives impressions gathered by the senses. Memory.

**Mantra**: Aid to meditation to help bring balance and stillness to the mind so that serenity and joy will prevail.

**Matrika Shakti**: The subtle vibrations of consciousness that arise as thoughts in the mind. These thoughts bring into awareness worlds that do not exist and are the fundamental illusion of life. Everything we think is wrong; the words that represent what is real, are not it.

**Maya**: The principle of creative illusion. Fascination with the thought constructs ever emerging in the mind. The veil over reality.

**Mayiya Mala**: The sense of differentiation. The belief that the consciousness that looks out of my eyes is different than the consciousness that sees through your eyes.

**Mudra**: 1. Attitude of the body or hand, as in a spontaneous yogic postures. 2. State of consciousness, as in kechari mudra, or mudra virya.

**Nirvana**: Buddha Nature, cessation of thought, purity, perfection.

**Nirvikalpa**: Thought-free state.

**Niyama**: Observance of purification, contentment, scriptural study, mantra repetition, austerity and devotion.

**Noumena**: Intangible essence.

**Paramashiva**: Quintessence of the first cause.

**Prakasha**: Principle of self-revelation, or light of illumination by which everything is known; light of consciousness and source of intelligence. Prakasha lies beyond the mind as the witness to the appearance and knower of the thoughts. It is revealed when the mind is utterly still, as the experience of just being.

**Pralaya**: Great sleep of consciousness between epochs of universal manifestation.

**Prana**: Breath of life.

**Pranayama**: Yogic breath practice to clear the mind, increase vital capacity, purify circulation and vitalize organ systems.

**Puja**: 1. Devotional altar. 2. Ceremony of reverence.

**Rajas**: Guna, or quality, of stimulation and activity.

**Sadhana**: Practice of spiritual discipline; meditation, devotion, scriptural study, satsang, darshan.

**Samadhi**: State of unwavering calmness; with thought (savikalpa), or without thought (nirvikalpa).

**Samskara**: Impressions left in the mind after any experience; predisposition from past impressions.

**Satsang**: The company of devotees.

**Sattva**: Quality of purity, goodness and joy.

**Satya**: Truth.

**Seva**: Selfless service.

**Shakti**: The power of manifestation, action, awareness and Self-knowledge inherent in the first cause (Paramashiva).

**Shaktipat**: Spiritual awakening, transmission of grace usually given by a fully realized master of meditation.

**Shunyavidya**: Inner focus.

**Siddha**: Perfected being; free from the causal plane and effects of karma. A Siddha's state is infinite, pure and unlimited bliss.

**Spanda**: Unstruck universal vibration, resonating since the beginning of time. Audible as nada, the inner sound, in deep meditation.

**Tamas**: Guna, or quality of inertia.

**Tantra**: Philosophy and practice of attaining Self-realization through awakening of Kundalini Shakti.

**Vedanta**: Spiritual philosophy and practice rooted in the Vedas; specifically the Vedic Upanishads.

**Vimarsha**: Consciousness is understood in two aspects: Prakasha (light of awareness,) and Vimarsha (power of consciousness to know itself).

**Vimarshamaya**: Power (Mayashakti) of Vimarsha to differentiate the knower from the known.

**Vritti**: A mental process of objectification that mediates consciousness to its known object.

**Yoga**: There are five primary disciplines of Yoga: Hatha Yoga is the practice of postures (asanas) and breath control for health benefit. Karma Yoga is a life of righteous action following the observances and restraints (yamas and niyamas) given in the scriptures. Bhakti Yoga is a path of love and devotion toward a chosen deity or teacher (guru). Tantra Yoga awakens the power (kundalini) of spiritual Self-realization through the subtle energy channels (nadis) in the body. Jnana Yoga is the attainment of liberation through right understanding of the scriptures. There are also integrative yogas that practice all the primary paths (margas) as a comprehensive process to attain liberation (moksha), such as Raja Yoga and Siddha Yoga.